Before It Got

Complicated

Endorsements

"Bringing medical service to a city or region is a challenging effort, and recounting the history of that effort in Fort Smith and vicinity is not easy either. However, Taylor Prewitt . . . excels at research, and he is skillful at weaving all that information into an interesting and important work of medical history."

—*Tom Dillard*, writer on Arkansas history

"Taylor Prewitt . . . looks back to a simple time when people mattered in what could be termed the Camelot of medicine in Fort Smith. It's a great read and addition to the library of Fort Smith history."

—*Judge Jim Spears*, author and historian

"*Before It Got Complicated*—Every city and region should be so lucky as to have a dedicated scholar and physician like Taylor Prewitt to document their history."

—*Sam Taggart*, retired family physician and author

"I thoroughly enjoyed Dr. Prewitt's book on the rich history of medical practice in Fort Smith. Particularly noteworthy is the section on Dr. Harry McDonald . . . a fervent community activist who championed equality during the era of segregation."

—*George B. McGill*, mayor, Fort Smith

"Prewitt's eye for detail, summary of important people and events, and passion for a neglected area of local history, results in a book full of significant and interesting stories."

—*Tom Wing*. assistant professor of history, University of Arkansas-Fort Smith

"This work is a valuable addition to the bibliography of Arkansas medical history."

—*Timothy G. Nutt*, Director, Historical Research Center, University of Arkansas for Medical Sciences (UAMS) Library

"Prewitt has captured historical facts by way of being an engaging storyteller."

—*Lynn Wasson*, founding editor, Entertainment Fort Smith.

"Each chapter of "stories too good to keep" reveals the characters who had major roles, with their humor and tragedies, and the drama of healthcare as it unfolded here."

—*Billy D. Higgins*, emeritus associate professor of history, University of Arkansas-Fort Smith

Before It Got Complicated

Medicine in Fort Smith
and the Arkansas River Valley, 1817-1975

Taylor Prewitt

Red Engine Press
Fort Smith, Arkansas

Cover Design by Joyce Faulkner

Library of Congress Control Number: 2023945595

ISBN: 978-0-9885891-8-6 (softcover)

ISBN: 978-0-9885891-9-3 (hardcover)

RED ENGINE
PRESS

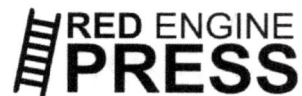

Born of the sun, they travelled a short while toward the sun.
And left the vivid air signed with their honour.

"I think continually of those who were truly great" – Stephen Spender

Table of Contents

Preface

To pass the time for my good friend and colleague, Leon Woods, in the last weeks of his terminal illness, his daughter Julie read him a few chapters of a collection of book reviews in the literature of medicine that I had recently written. Julie was at that time planning a series of programs at the Clayton House about the history of Fort Smith, so she asked me to present a Sunday afternoon talk on the history of medicine in this area. I assembled some of this information into a couple of papers that the *Journal of the Arkansas Medical Society* included in its 2013 issues.

It was about this time that my friend J.P. Bell invited me to join him on a field trip to Paris, Arkansas, where his medical school classmate, J.C. Smith, would show us the abandoned hospital that his grandfather and great uncle had built in 1913. J.P., by that time a well-known professional photographer, captured images in the dim light of the building that had hardly been touched since closing its doors in 1971. This experience we recorded in another paper for the *Journal of the Arkansas Medical Society*, telling the story of the three generations of rugged pioneer doctors who had practiced in Paris.

These projects generated momentum for a series of papers for the *Journal of the Fort Smith Historical Society*, presenting chapters from the history of medicine in western Arkansas and Fort Smith. One of these essays, "'He Knew Who He Was': Reflections on the Life and Mission of Harry P. McDonald," received the Walter L. Brown Award for Best Biography, Autobiography, or Memoir in a county or local journal, presented by the Arkansas Historical Association in 2018.

Adding a couple of chapters to fill in some of the corners, these pieces add up to a story line that joins the various subplots into the history of medicine in western Arkansas up to the 1970s, when things did begin to become complex.

One is tempted to refer to this segment of the past as a heroic saga, but we all know that heroism comes in many shades. Health care has never been simple, and as a human endeavor it's been the stuff of achievement and failure, motives good and bad, huge problems, a few successes, and a lot of hard work. In this collection of stories, we see developments like those that have happened over and over, in all corners of this country, for years and years. This happens to be what I have learned about this place and these people. These stories are too good to keep.

—Taylor Prewitt

Introduction

The President of the United States came to Fort Smith on August 10, 1975, to dedicate the newly relocated St. Edward Mercy Medical Center on the east side of town, at the corner of Rogers Avenue and Seventy-fourth Street. St. Edward had previously been located downtown at Rogers and Lexington. Sparks Regional Medical Center, south of downtown and soon to become for a short time the largest hospital in Arkansas with an expansion in 1979, occupied the other magnetic pole of medical care.

And on this day, with President Gerald Ford in attendance, the shape of medical care in Fort Smith changed. It got complicated.

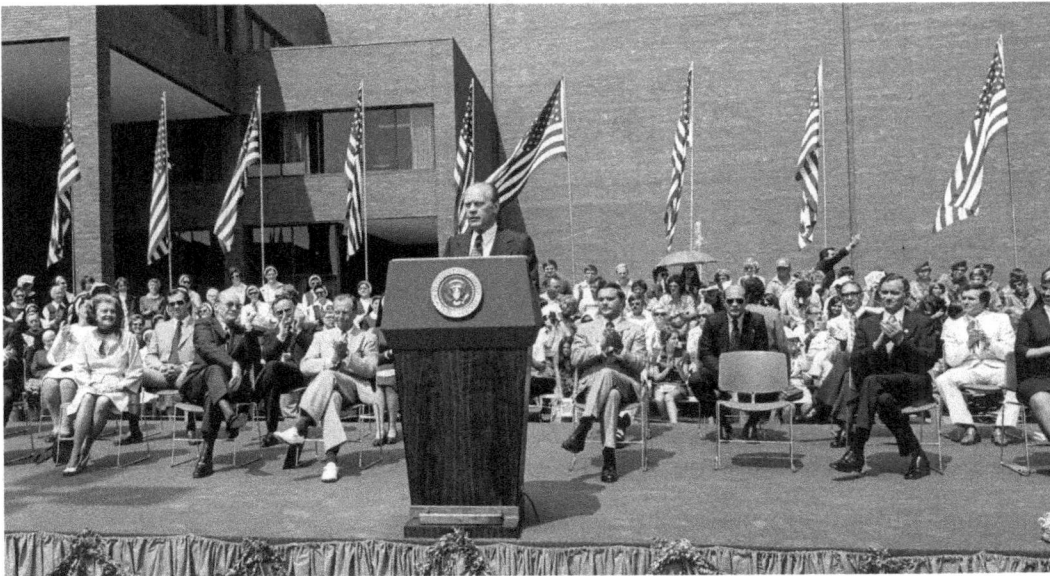

President Gerald Ford dedicates the new St. Edward Hospital on August 10, 1975, ushering in a new era in health care delivery. (Mercy Fort Smith archives)

Of course, President Ford's appearance in 1975 had nothing to do with the arc of medical history in this region. But it marks a convenient punctuation point for the scope of this book, covering the years between the establishment of medical care in the original fort in 1817, when things were simple, and the stretching of hospital care to the eastern reaches of the city in 1975, when there was a certain loss of innocence with new layers of complexity.

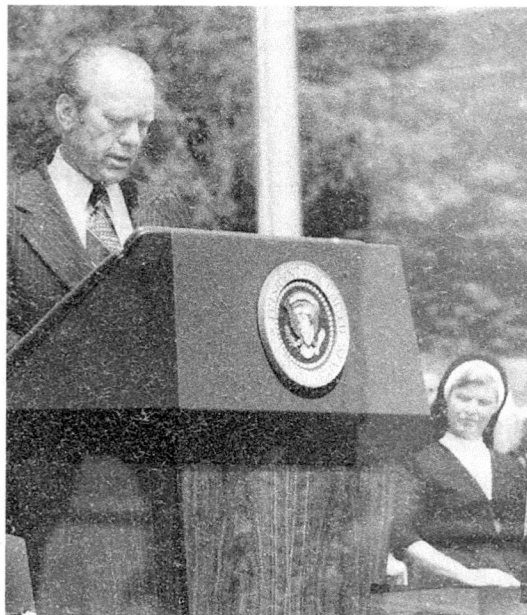

Sister Judith Marie Keith, administrator of St. Edward Hospital, looks on as President Ford speaks at the dedication ceremony. (Mercy Fort Smith archives)

Things have always been complicated, of course; it's just a matter of degree. But few will disagree that medical care nowadays is really complicated. The passage of time allows us the opportunity to view developments in the long run, tracing the major trends to see how it began to get this way.

Variations of these events have played out in one form or another all over the country during the same time. But the devil is in the details, and zeroing in on the hills and prairies and valleys of western Arkansas, with the urban focal point of Fort Smith, helps us to focus back and forth between the details and the big picture.

Three stages of development help us to trace this history. They may overlap a bit, but the first stage may be allotted to the nineteenth century, with development of professionalism in private medical practice. Lone physicians and small groups realized the importance of keeping up to date—and of persuading the public that they were doing so, by various means of certification to obtain credibility.

It was the second stage of development, already beginning after the end of the Civil War, that brought real advances in quality of life and life expectancy. This was the time of public health improvements, extending beyond the scope of private practice. Muddy streets were paved, outdoor privies were replaced with indoor plumbing, water became safer to drink, better food supply brought improved nutrition, vaccines were developed, and some dent was made in the population of disease-bearing mosquitoes.

Two specific diseases posed major challenges to this system of public and private health care. One was a chronic disease that exacted a continual toll: tuberculosis. The other was a short-lived disaster that struck like a prairie fire and subsided in a relatively short time: influenza, in the form of a worldwide pandemic that totally disrupted the life of the community as it claimed more American lives in three months than all the wars of the twentieth century.

Tuberculosis was fought with a sanatorium system; influenza, with ad-hoc policies of isolation and hygiene.

In the wake of the influenza pandemic and the end of the Great War, Fort Smith was the site of a third development that anticipated a national phenomenon that took place a few decades later: the coming together of individual medical practices into group practices that became progressively larger. Inspired by the example of the newly named (1914) Mayo Clinic, St. Cloud Cooper organized Cooper Clinic in 1920, followed only a few months later by the formation of a similar multi-specialty clinic by Charles Holt. Fred Krock joined him a few years later, and Holt-Krock Clinic soon became, for a time, the largest private group practice in Arkansas.

America was still in the throes of the Jim Crow era in mid-century. As the civil rights movement began to awaken the country to the gratuitous cruelties of racism, segregated wards in hospitals, and even segregated hospitals, began to disappear. Young African-American men and women began, with courage and determination, to enter the healing professions in greater numbers. This revolution is reflected in the story of Dr. Harry P. McDonald, who came to Fort Smith with a conscious mission to be an agent of change. One lifetime wasn't enough to do everything that needed to be done, but his accomplishments illustrate the changes that have taken place in this country in the space of a couple of generations.

Times were changing.

The complicated events of the last four decades are a story for another day. But even the most complex stories start somewhere. In this part of the United States, the story began in 1817.

The First Hundred Years 1820-1920

A Hospital in the Fort

A hospital occupied a portion of the small frontier fort erected by Major William Bradford after he and his sixty-four men arrived at Belle Point on Christmas Day, 1817. Four were seriously ill and six were convalescent when they arrived, but on New Year's Day, 1818, Major Bradford wrote, "I have them all comfortably situated together with a hospital for the sick. . ." [1]

Thus began the activities of the first hospital in Arkansas, at the time of the founding of Fort Smith. There was no doctor at "Camp Smith"—named after Rifle Regiment Commander Thomas A. Smith—until Dr. Thomas Russell, Surgeon, United States Army, arrived later in 1818. Dr. Russell's tenure was brief; he died at the fort of a "nervous fever" in August 1819, and he is thought to have been the first person buried in the site now known as the National Cemetery. [2, 3]

The hospital at Fort Smith was busy from the first: sometimes as many as twenty percent of the seventy enlisted men were hospitalized or kept in the barracks, most due to "ague and bilious fever." Malaria and yellow fever were raging at this time, and the following account by Thomas Nuttall describes their effects:

> From July to October, the ague and bilious fever spread throughout the territory in a very unusual manner. Connected apparently with these diseases, was one of an extraordinary character. It commenced by slight chills, and was succeeded by a fever, attended with unremitting vomiting, accompanied with blood, and bloody foeces (sic). Ejecting all medicine, it became next to impossible to administer internal relief. The paroxysms, attended with excruciating pain, took place every other day, similar to the common intermittent. One of the soldiers who descended with us, was afflicted in this way for the space of six days, after which he recovered. On the intermitting days he appeared perfectly easy and possessed a strong and craving appetite. I was credibly informed that not less than one hundred of the Cherokees, settled contiguous to the banks of the Arkansa, (sic) died this season of the bilious fever. [4]

Significant improvement in health conditions at this time were more often due to public health measures than to individual medical care, and health in the fort began to improve with the planting of gardens and the raising of crops and livestock. The post hospital again had a surgeon in 1823, Richard M. Coleman.

Remedies were limited—calomel, castor oil, a tonic of Peruvian bark, mustard and linseed plasters, and frequent bloodletting, either surgical or with leeches. Recruits to the army were screened for tumors, ulcerated legs, rupture, skin infections, and piles. All who had not had smallpox were vaccinated. Fifty men at Fort Smith died of yellow fever in 1823. [5]

Movement of the troops to Fort Towson and Fort Gibson left the fort unoccupied from 1824 to 1833, but a civilian population had been established in the town. Assistant Surgeon C.B. Welch reported a host of rather unhealthy conditions in 1834—bilious fever, enlarged spleen, ascites, anasarca, pneumonia, pleuritis, diarrhea, chronic enteritis, and a wide variety of other derangements of the liver and gastrointestinal tract. Eight soldiers and one assistant surgeon died. [6]

A new fort was constructed from 1838 to 1843. Assistant Surgeon William Hammond agreed to care for the civilian construction workers in addition to the troops, but he found the post hospital wanting in amenities: two "very indifferent apartments," with one window but no sash or glass—an "old dilapidated building in a half falling condition" with no benches, tables, bunks, or kitchen. [7] There were, however, civilian doctors: Dr. Joseph Bailey, who had been with the army in Fort Smith in 1836; Dr. J.D. McGee in Van Buren; and Dr. J.H.T. Main, hired by the fort commander to care for the construction workers.

Standards of health care lagged at the fort, and a visiting general in 1845 reported that there were no provisions for care of the sick. His orders led to renovation of some of the officers' quarters as a hospital with additional space for a surgeon. An undiagnosed illness called "the cold plague" struck the fort in the winter of 1846, afflicting half the troops, of whom several died. Ordinary funeral procedures were curtailed for fear of their having an adverse effect on the soldiers' morale. [8]

With a measure of prosperity and growth, Fort Smith was able to retain physicians. Dr. Main stayed for the rest of his life, and Dr. Bailey remained as post surgeon for many years. Dr. W.W. Bailey married the daughter of Dr. Main, and the home that Dr. Main built for the young couple was later occupied by Holt-Krock Clinic at the corner of Lexington and Dodson Avenues from 1953 to 1979. [9]

Private practices began to grow: two physicians, Dr. S.H. Payne and Dr. W.F. Blakemore, began practice in Greenwood in the early 1850s; and the 1860 business directory of Fort Smith listed six physicians: J.H.T. Main, N. Spring, E.R. DuVal, J.E. Bromford, William Beall, and A.S. Dunlap.

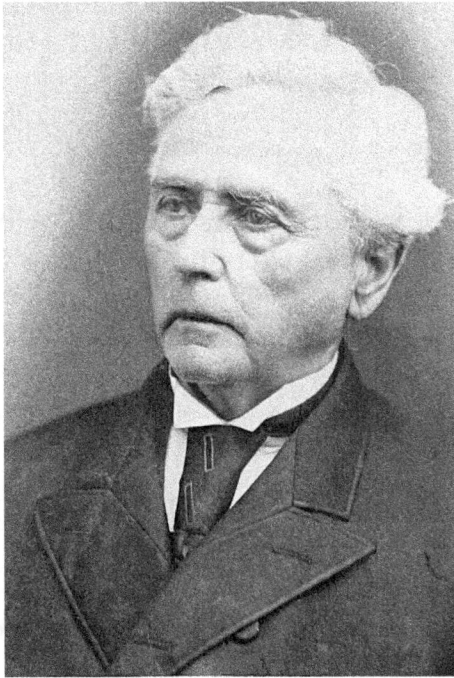

J. H. T. Main (1813-1891) came to Fort Smith in the 1830s as a physician to the Army and remained to become the first civilian physician in Fort Smith. [1]

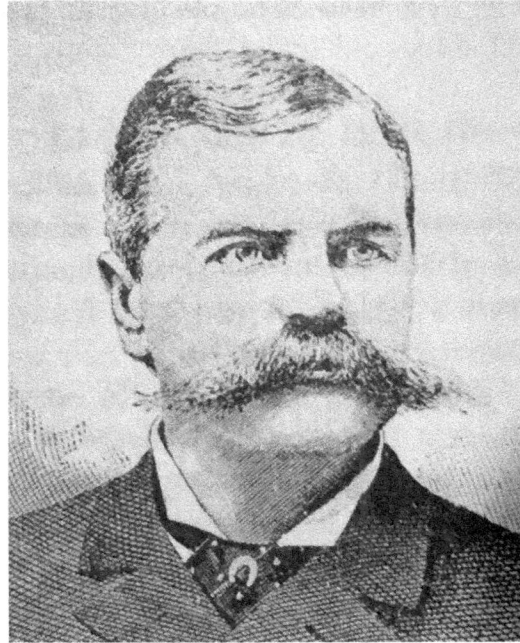

William Worth Bailey, son-in-law of Dr. J. H. T. Main, was the first chief of staff of St. John's Hospital. [1]

Of these, Dr. Nicholas Spring was mayor of Fort Smith in 1850. He and his brother-in-law William Sutton operated a mercantile business, Sutton and Spring, which was one of thirteen businesses destroyed by a fire in 1860. Their business lost $40,000, and Sutton, who had built the house now known as the Clayton House, lost $12,000. Sutton abandoned his house and fled to Texas as the Civil War began. The house then became one of six buildings comprising the U.S. General Hospital, maintained by Union forces after they occupied Fort Smith in 1863. [10]

Before the fort's hospital closed, it played a part in the treatment of African Americans. The black soldiers of the 11th U.S. Colored Infantry were treated at the U.S. General Hospital, as the hospital at the fort became known. There was a sequence of names for this institution: the Military Hospital, the Colored Military Hospital, the Colored Hospital of Fort Smith, and the Freedman's Hospital. For several days after Appomattox the city was under the direct patrol of the black soldiers of the 57th U.S. Colored Infantry. The Freedman's Hospital served the refugee population, which was white, as well as the Freedmen. [11]

In a city with a population of 2,227 in 1870, the most frequent diseases were yellow fever, dysenteries, and malaria. [12] Dr. Spring and Dr. Main offered free care to the families of Confederate veterans.

Good Health Begins at Home

Medical care in the nineteenth century began at home. Doctors had offices (often in their own homes), but they routinely went to the homes of the sick, who were often unable to leave the bed, and perhaps more often reluctant to do so. If surgery was indicated, it too was performed in the patient's home as a matter of course. Civilian hospitals began to appear late in the century; these were initially for those who lacked the resources for home care, but gradually hospitals began to provide private rooms and other amenities for paying patients.

What operations were done in the home? Not just the little stuff. Under a headline, "OPERATED FOR GALL STONES", the Fort Smith *Southwest American* reported on July 26, 1908, "Mrs. Mary C. Kayser was operated on for gall stones at her residence near the Electric Park, and was relieved of about eighteen stones, some of which are as large as ordinary marbles. The technique of the operation was rendered very difficult by the extensive adhesions which during the protracted period of her illness had formed between the under surface of the liver and the adjacent coils of intestine, in the deep recesses of which the stones were lodged. This was the fourth cholecystectomy Dr. Jules Ludeau had done, all in private residences, and all four made a rapid recovery." [13]

Surgeons sometimes traveled near and far to perform home surgery. Dr. Marlin Hoge, a retired surgeon in Fort Smith, recalled accompanying his father to Ozark, Arkansas, some forty miles east of Fort Smith, to perform surgery at rural farmhouses in the 1920s and 1930s, even though his Fort Smith surgery was done in one of the hospitals. Dr. St. Cloud Cooper, founder of Cooper Clinic, drove the twenty-four miles from Fort Smith to Sallisaw, Oklahoma, to remove her mother's gall bladder in her home, one of my patients told me. Records of the Sebastian County Medical Society indicate that Dr. Cooper presented a program on the gall bladder and its surgery at one of its meetings in 1907. [14]

It was claimed that kitchen surgery allowed avoidance of hospital-borne infections, if the operator could keep his own hands clean. Rubber gloves came along a little later, but rapid surgery was emphasized to decreases the time of exposure. Instruments were to be kept away from the unwashed skin and were always to be put back into the dishpan after use. [15]

Preparations included boiling the instruments, removing furniture and pictures, scrubbing the walls and floor, and nailing sheets on the windows to keep the neighbors from peeping in. [16] With the advent of the automobile, a car could sometimes be driven up to the window of the room to be used for surgery. Someone could be delegated to hold up a mirror to deflect the light from the car's headlights onto the operative field. In one account, an appendectomy was done using light from a headlight detached from the car and connected to the gas tank by a rubber hose running through the window of the kitchen. [17]

House calls persisted longer than kitchen surgery. Curiously, the migration of patient care from home to hospital, clinic, and office is remembered more widely for the almost complete disappearance of the house call than for the abandonment of kitchen surgery. I think that the perception increased that little could be done in the home, and that proper management required a visit to an urgent care center or an emergency room or a doctor's office.

Dr. St. Cloud Cooper's notebook, given to me by his granddaughter, lists his house calls from 1920 until his death in 1930. As one example, during the week of June 4-10, 1920, Dr. Cooper made seven house calls on Sunday, seven on Monday, eleven on Tuesday, eight on Wednesday, ten on Thursday, eight on Friday, and nine on Saturday. What could Dr. Cooper do on a 1920 house call, with limited resources? Here is one answer: "First of all, the physician was expected to walk in and take over; he became responsible for the outcome whether he could affect it or not. Second, it was assumed that he would stand by, on call, until it was over. Third, and this was probably the most important of his duties, he would explain what had happened and what was likely to happen." [18]

Dr. Henry Hollenberg of Little Rock emphasized that in the absence of hospitals in 1875, everyone was treated at home; a household was expected to know how to set up sick quarters for treatment of the common and dreaded pneumonia, typhoid fever and the often-fatal dysenteries. [19]

Dr. William Duncan of Arkansas elaborated on the contents of the doctor's bag: "Every doctor carried a goodly supply of English Calomel, some aloes, and Dover's powder. Opium, in some form or another, sweet Spirits of Nitre, a preparation of Spanish Fly for drawing blisters, and in districts where ague was prevalent, Peruvian Bark constituted an essential of his material medica. Sulphate of quinine was yet too rare and costly for general use in practice. As bloodletting was considered of first importance in cases of malignant fever, he carried one or more lancets to be ready for any emergency." [20]

Before the advent of the automobile, doctors traveled on horseback and by horse and buggy. Since it is generally known that doctors drive too fast, one wonders how fast they could go. One country doctor gave this estimate: "Seven miles an hour was good time in cold weather with good roads; three miles was customary on muddy roads; and a mule would walk two and a half miles an hour if unmolested. If urged, however, he would slow down to two miles an hour, and if urged too much he would stop completely and look back over his shoulder to ask what you were going to do about it." [21]

Cleaning Things Up

Discovery of gold at Sutter's Mill in California in 1848 led to the Gold Rush, and Fort Smith became a major jumping-off place, with as many as three hundred people in Fort Smith in March 1849, waiting for a time to start. This was not an unmixed blessing; when the steamboat *Robert Morris* arrived in Fort Smith on the evening of April 15, several of the crew and passengers, including two pilots, had died of cholera. Surprisingly, this did not lead to a local epidemic, although there were several cases of cholera in an emigrant camp four miles from town. The newspaper called for cleansing the city, saying that any inspection of the city would "find dead carcasses and filth, of various kinds, enough to produce pestilence." A freeze with several inches of snow on April 14 and 15 probably helped spare Fort Smith from a cholera epidemic this time. In 1851, however, cholera did strike the city, with many deaths. Dr. W.H. Mayers of No. 1, Commercial Row, capitalized on this outbreak by marketing his "Cholera preparation," demonstrating its efficacy by publicly administering it to a man "who was suffering with the diarrhea," with a report of immediate relief. [22]

Editor John F. Wheeler of the Fort Smith *Herald* proved to be a crusader for cleaning up the city, and he chaired a meeting at "the church" (a building initially used by several denominations), where a three-man team was appointed to inspect the city's houses. Any who refused to cleanse their houses on orders from this committee were to be reported to the Town Council. The Council also ordered the cleaning of the streets and alleys and sprinkling them with lime.

Editor Wheeler appeared to be pleased with the results. In a newspaper article protesting the removal of the troops from Fort Smith to Fort Gibson, he stated:

> "A more healthy place for troops we venture to say, is not to be found in the United States than Fort Smith. During the time the two companies of the 5th Infantry were stationed here, which is nearly two years, there were not exceeding half a dozen deaths, including those brought here with disease, contracted while in Mexico. Not

a case of Cholera was among them last season, though the soldiers were called upon to remove freight from boats that had disease upon them." [23]

Despite these claims, the hot summer of 1850, with temperatures of 100–105, brought a smallpox epidemic, which ran its course through the end of August.

The prevailing diseases were pneumonia and smallpox; there were also forty cases of what was called "vaccination syphilis," spreading to 500–600 cases with all the symptoms of true syphilis. Syphilis was once thought to be transmitted by smallpox vaccination, an association no longer accepted, so one would suspect that syphilis was syphilis. As an example of the case load at the military hospital at Fort Smith, 263 patients were admitted during December 1863; of these, sixteen died, three deserted, and seventy-seven returned to duty. There were sixty-four cases of pneumonia, thirty-four of smallpox, and thirty-nine of "spurious vaccination"—probably syphilis. [24]

The city was damaged by the Civil War. Cemeteries were spoiled; "yard and garden fences have disappeared; fruit trees and shrubbery have been destroyed." The fort's hospital was abandoned in 1869, and indeed the fort itself closed in 1871. This was a time when mosquito-borne diseases were continuing to exact a heavy toll. There were eighty-two cases of malaria reported in the fort during the first eight months of 1869. Other illnesses were less numerous: five cases of dysentery, five of venereal disease, and three of rheumatism. There was one death. [25]

Fort Smith initiated more vigorous public health measures in the years after the Civil War. The city council appointed Dr. J.G. Eberle to try to overcome the numerous obstacles to improving the streets at a time when Garrison Avenue was described as "belly deep in mud." With the issuance of bonds that were without legal status, and without any laws to facilitate the collection of taxes, Dr. Eberle saw to it that the paving of the streets was begun in 1888 and completed in 1891. All the bonds were paid off in 1907. The soft red bricks used in the original paving lasted only twenty-three years, and wood blocks were laid in 1912–1913. When the wood warped, new brick paving was finally laid on Garrison in 1924, laid over the original 1888 five-inch concrete base. [26] By 1898 there was a "magnificent system of water works," with drains and sewers, sidewalks, and streetlamps. Boasting in 1891 of an "ideal climate, perfect sewer system, and pure water," the city claimed that its mortality rate of eighteen per thousand population was far below that of New Orleans—29.2 deaths per thousand. [27]

Mortality rates were a valid cause for concern in the nineteenth century. One of the greatest epidemics of our time had hit Memphis in 1878 when yellow fever struck. In a city where even the most well-bred ladies wore rubber boots down-town because of the mud, the biggest problem was that of raw sewage, and the privies were usually located less than fifty feet from drinking wells. The *Aedes Aegypti* mosquito, which transferred the virus from person to person, made its way in ships from Africa to Havana, then to New Orleans, and finally by steamboats up the Mississippi River to Memphis, where stagnant water was abundant. When it became known that yellow fever had appeared, more than half the city's population fled the city in a span of five days. The population of Memphis was 47,000 in July 1878. By September, 19,000 remained; 17,000 of them had yellow fever. Of these, 5,000 died. There were 20,000 deaths in the Mississippi River Valley. The heat was stifling that summer; the stench from the dead and the dying was said to be overwhelming. [28]

Arkansans were terrified, especially those in Little Rock and the eastern part of the state, but also as far west as Fort Smith. Mr. and Mrs. Alexander Hager vowed that if Little Rock were spared, they would devote their entire estate to the founding of a hospital, thus leading to the establishment of St. Vincent Infirmary in 1888. [29] And the newly formed Arkansas Medical Society (not the state legislature) formed the first state board of health in 1879 to enforce quarantine regulations to prevent the spread of yellow fever. The Legislature did indeed fund a state board of health in 1881, but after two years, in the absence of further spread of yellow fever, the appropriation was not renewed. [30]

Dr. J.A. Dibrell and the Quest for Legitimacy

The early 19th century was a time when medicine and society were feeling their way toward a system of providing health care without exposing the population to unscrupulous quacks. Some of the physicians in the territory persuaded the Arkansas Territorial Legislation to set up a licensing board for physicians in 1832; a state board of eight physicians would have had absolute power in granting licenses. However, the territorial governor, John Pope, thought the growing territory needed more, not fewer, doctors, and he vetoed the provision, saying that "the highest authority known in this land, public opinion," was superior to diplomas. [31]

Such legislation was not unusual at this time, with suspicion of entrenched elites attributed to the culture of Jacksonian America. "Many state legislatures in this era abolished all restrictions on who could become a doctor or a lawyer in order to discourage 'monopolies.'" [32]

Dr. J.A. Dibrell of Van Buren attempted unsuccessfully to organize a county medical society in 1845, to include the Fort Smith army physicians. [33] (This was before Sebastian County was split off from Crawford County in 1851.)

This far-seeing physician who conceived the idea of a medical society in Crawford County, James A. Dibrell, went on to have a distinguished career and to be the father of three physicians. He was only twenty-eight years old when he proposed a county medical society in 1845; three years later he was described in a newspaper article as a "colorful figure" who "looks taller than his five feet ten inches because of the stovepipe hat he often wears. With gray hair and hazel eyes, he carries a gold headed, engraved walking cane." He was "one of very few trained physicians [who] often travels long distances on horseback into the Ozark Mountains and to the Indian Territory to treat patients," as told in the Doctors Hall of Honor in the Arkansas Country Doctor Museum in Lincoln, Arkansas. [34]

Dr. Dibrell oversaw the wounded Confederate soldiers after the Battle of Prairie Grove. He moved his family to Little Rock for safety, and he was then drafted as a surgeon for the Union Army after it took Little Rock.

James A. Dibrell, Jr. had to earn his college expenses because his father lost all his holdings in the war. After earning his medical degree in 1870, he settled in Little Rock, and in 1879 he was one of eight incorporators of a medical school for the University of Arkansas, known as the Medical Department of Arkansas Industrial University, now the University of Arkansas for Medical Sciences. Dr. Dibrell Jr. was professor of anatomy and in 1886 became president of the faculty, then serving as the dean until his death of pneumonia in 1904 at age fifty-eight. His two sons, John and James (grandsons of James Dibrell, Sr.), both became physicians and members of the faculty. [35]

Dr. Dibrell Sr. had two other sons who became physicians: Edwin, who practiced in Little Rock, and Matt, who returned to Van Buren to practice. Dr. Matt Dibrell made calls with a horse (named Harvey) and buggy, then in a surrey with a fringe on top, and finally in a four-cylinder Buick. Of the four daughters of Dr. Dibrell, Sr., two married physicians—Dr. Elias DuVal of Fort Smith and Dr. George Hynes of Fort Smith. One of the other two daughters, Ann Eliza, married George Sparks of Fort Smith. She died early, and as described below, Sparks Hospital was named in her memory in accordance with a stipulation in a bequest to the hospital by her husband George Sparks.

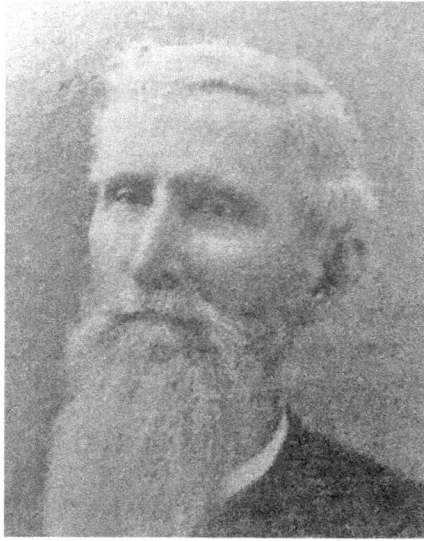

James A. Dibrell, Sr., of Van Buren initiated the first county medical society in the state in 1845, two years before the formation of the American Medical Association. (Photo from Arkansas Country Doctors Museum)

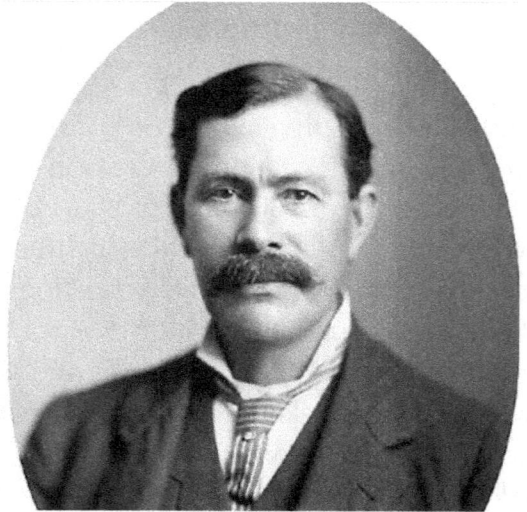

Dr. James Dibrell, Jr., was one of the founders of the University of Arkansas School of Medicine in 1879. (Photo from Encyclopedia of Arkansas)

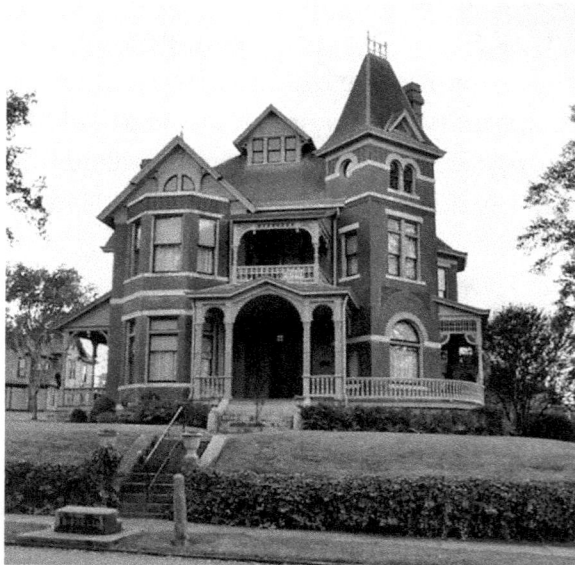

The James A. Dibrell House, still in use as a private residence at 1400 Spring Street in Little Rock, was known for being up to date with the latest innovations. (Photo by author)

After the death of Dr. Dibrell Sr. in 1897 at age eighty, his funeral was "one of the largest ever seen in western Arkansas" with all businesses in Van Buren closed. He was buried in Fairview Cemetery in Van Buren. [36]

Two years after Dr. Dibrell's initial attempt to organize the physicians of Crawford County in 1845, the American Medical Association was organized to address the issue of lax standards for physicians and to separate the "regular from the irregular practitioners" such as homeopaths, to be distinguished from "allopaths" who practiced regular medicine. [37]

The Medical Association of the state of Arkansas held an organizational meeting in 1870, attended by Drs. E.R. DuVal and J.C. Field of Fort Smith, representing Sebastian County. However, this society disbanded in 1875 after exhausting its resources in dealing with a dispute in which one Hot Springs physician filed charges against another. [38] The society was solving this problem by dissolving itself and reorganizing in the same year under a new name, the Arkansas Medical Society, with basically the same membership (without, one would hope, the two disputatious Hot Springs physicians).

Sixteen doctors from Sebastian and Crawford Counties were among the charter members when the Arkansas Medical Society obtained its charter on October 11, 1875. Six of these had been charter members of the Sebastian County Medical Society. A list of their names and the medical schools they had attended shows a diversity of backgrounds: W. Worth Bailey, University of Michigan; J.E. Bennett, University of Maryland; J.W. Breedlove, University of Louisville; Albert Dunlap, Transylvania University; Elias R. DuVal, Pennsylvania Medical College; and J.H.T. Main, Sterling Medical College, Columbus, Ohio. [39]

The Sebastian County doctors had already organized during this time, forming the Sebastian County Medical Society at Greenwood (then the county seat) on March 2, 1874, with fifteen physicians. This society designated itself as an auxiliary of the state society, and it adopted the Code of Ethics of the American Medical Association (AMA). Its objects were to enable the members of the profession "to keep pace with the progressive spirit of the age in which we live; to promote peace and concord among its members; and to engender a love of science." A candidate for membership was required to demonstrate good moral character, to have graduated from a medical school recognized by the AMA, and to have received no more than two blackballs.

Some members of the society objected to the application of Dr. J. Price because he had circulated "unethical cards" listing a change in his "individual" fees. There was sensitivity about some "irregular" physicians attempting to attract patients with low fees, and there was some discussion of setting a standardized list of fees. This idea was rejected, however, and it was agreed that fees would be "individually determined." And so, Dr. Price was admitted to membership.

Other "doctors" were more irregular. For instance, the Fort Smith *Elevator* reported in 1880 that Dr. Preston was continuing to entertain crowds of listeners on the Avenue with his comic songs as he discussed the merits of his famous worm medicine. The new county medical society was not amused, and in 1883 its Judicial Committee reported that no members of the regular profession were to consult with the "irregulars." The issue of fees did not die, and later in this same year eleven physicians of the county society signed a fee list in hopes that it would place the members of the society above reproach in the matter of commercialism. An ordinary visit was $2. A few of the other fees were: $10 for syphilis (to be paid in advance); $50–$100 for a strangulated hernia; and $5–$50 for hemorrhoids.

A certain Dr. Kelleam was removed from the society in 1892 for advertising specific treatments. Four standards were established: advertising a specialty or treatment of one disease was forbidden; placing cards in public was acceptable but not encouraged; "irregulars" were to be consulted only in an emergency; and consultation with regular physicians was to be done in the most professional manner. [40]

The Sebastian County Medical Society was among the earliest to admit a woman. This was Dr. Minnie Sanders, educated at Union Academy in Anna, Illinois; Woman's Medical College in St. Louis; Woman's College in Chicago (later Rush Medical College); and Keokuk Medical School in Iowa, from which she received her medical degree in 1890. She became a demonstrator in anatomy at Woman's Medical College in St. Louis and assistant to the chair of gynecology there. She practiced with her father in Jonesboro, Illinois, where she was called to jury duty. A physician was required for a particular case, and no male doctor could be located. Accordingly, the judge declared her to be a "person" and allowed her to serve, becoming perhaps the first woman juror in the world.

She came to Fort Smith at the invitation of her cousin, Mrs. W.P. Throgmorton, wife of the pastor of the First Baptist Church, thinking that her poor health would be improved in a milder climate. She practiced from 1892 to 1895, when she retired to marry Henry Clay Armstrong. [41] She bore four children, including Minnie Ruth Armstrong, a public-school teacher for whom the Ruth Armstrong Nature Area at Old Greenwood and Rogers Avenue is named.

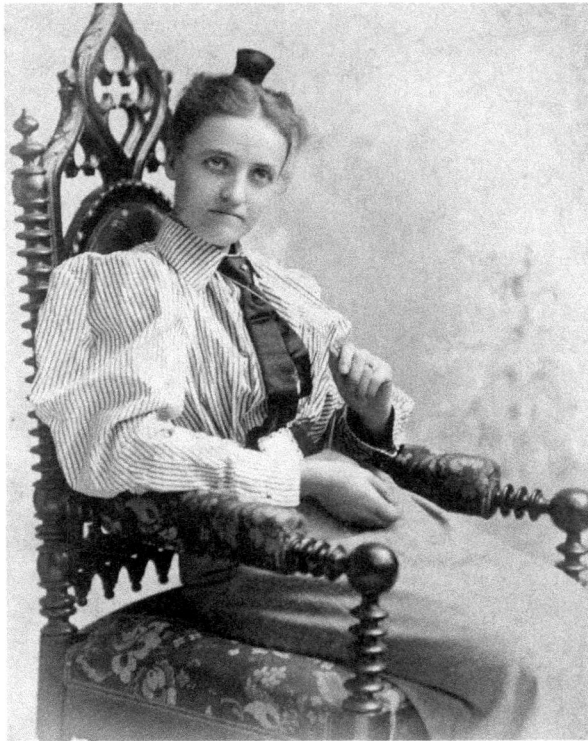

Minnie Sanders (1867-1956) was the first woman physician in Fort Smith, where she practiced from 1892 to 1895. She retired to marry Henry Clay Armstrong. (Photo courtesy of Missy Roebuck)

Treating Patients in a Hospital

A railroad employee crushed his foot while at work one day in 1887 in Fort Smith. It soon became infected, requiring amputation, but he had no friends and no funds. A physician was willing to operate without a fee, but surgery was usually done in the home, and he was an itinerant worker without a place where the surgery could be done. Rev. George Degen of St. John's Episcopal Church learned of this dilemma and raised $500 to rent a vacant building at Fourth and G Streets. The women of the church supplied furniture and linens, and the patient and physician moved into this new "hospital," which became known as St. John's Hospital, the first civilian hospital in Arkansas. [42] (The 1883–84 Fort Smith City Directory listed "The Fort Smith Hospital and Free Dispensary—Hospital, Mulberry at the corner of Howard." There are no further records of this hospital, or when it closed.) [43] A women's volunteer group kept St. John's open, and it was incorporated by the state in 1890, with Federal Judge Isaac C. Parker as the first president of the board of trustees.

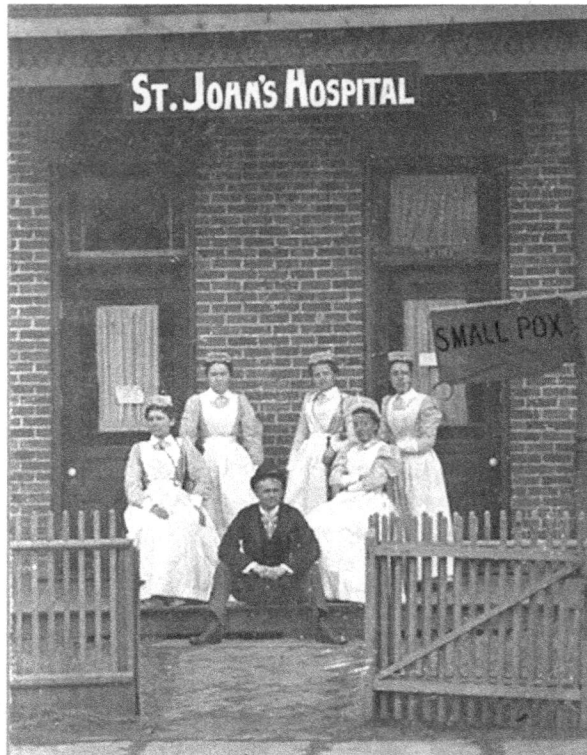

St. John's Hospital was organized in 1887; during the 1890s it was located at Fourth and Oak Streets, the apparent site of this photograph of a physician and nurses during the time of a smallpox epidemic. (Photo courtesy of Fort Smith Museum of History)

Staff physicians were elected by the county medical society, with Dr. W.W. Bailey as the first chief of staff. A crisis occurred when a group of "irregular" physicians, the Progressive Medical Society, insisted on their right to admit patients. The medical society responded that charity patients could be admitted only with the approval of the chief of staff or a visiting physician (all members of the county society). No patients of "irregulars" could be admitted. Here the board of trustees intervened and ruled that one third of the hospital could be controlled by the Progressive Medical Society. The county medical society found this unacceptable; they withdrew from St. John's and organized a City Charity Hospital. In the end, the two hospitals were united to form the Belle Point Hospital, and the Progressive Medical Society ceased to exist. This hospital moved to a new building on 916 South Twelfth Street in 1902, and in 1908 George T. Sparks, a member of the board of trustees, left $25,000 to the hospital with the condition that it be named Sparks Hospital in memory of his wife, Ann Eliza Dibrell Sparks, a daughter of Dr. James A. Dibrell of Van Buren. [44]

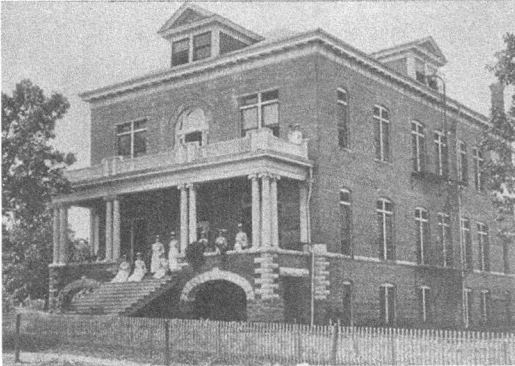

Belle Point Hospital was formed in 1899 by the merger of St. John's and City Charity Hospitals. This photograph is dated about 1902, the year the hospital moved from North Tenth and B Streets to a new building on 916 South Twelfth Street. (Photo courtesy of Fort Smith Museum of History)

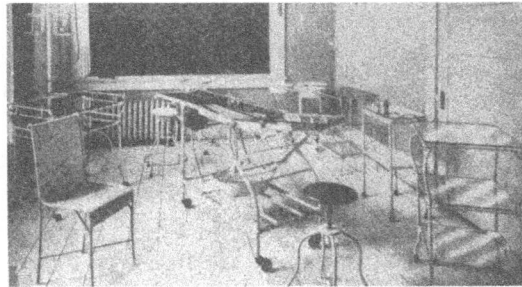

Surgery began to move from kitchen tables to the hospital in the late nineteenth and early twentieth centuries, as shown in this operating room at the Belle Point Hospital. Many patients preferred to have their surgery at home for several years. (Photo from [9])

(George Sparks was a grandson of Aaron Barling, who came to Fort Smith as a soldier in 1822 and stayed after his service ended in 1824. He purchased 450 acres of land at what is now Barling. In 1825 his wife traveled by boat from Baltimore to New Orleans, thence up the river to Fort Smith.)

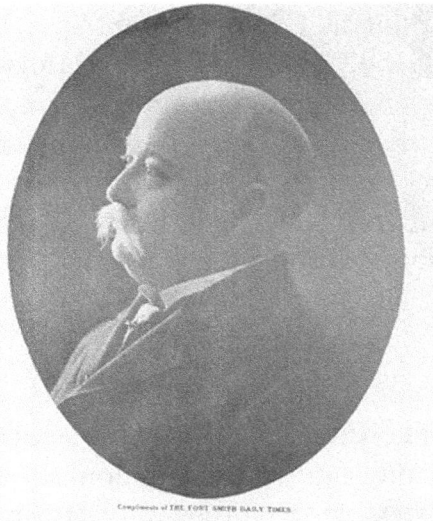

George T. Sparks (Photo courtesy of Fort Smith Museum of History)

The Sparks bequest allowed the hospital to add a new wing, increasing its capacity to one hundred beds. Paying patients were now willing to leave home to enter the hospital, which had been primarily a refuge for those unable to pay. Sparks did maintain two charity wards, with a ten-bed annex for African Americans.

St. John's Hospital established Arkansas's first nursing school in 1895, graduating its first class of three young women in 1898; and by 1914 there were fourteen hospitals in the state offering nursing courses. The Arkansas State Nurses' Association was organized in 1912, and in the following year the legislature passed a law that prevented unqualified nurses from calling themselves "registered." [45]

More hospitals continued to crop up. Jules Ludeau grew up in Louisiana, received his medical degree in Kentucky, and moved to Fort Smith in 1906 and opened the Fort Smith Medical Institute. He built the Ludeau Hospital in 1910, also known as the Fort Smith Hospital, at 1425 North Eleventh Street. This he sold in 1913 to Dr. Charles Holt and Dr. A.J. Morrisey, who changed its name to St. John's Hospital. (This is rather confusing. The name "St. John's" had been used before for the original hospital opened in 1887 but later merged with City Charity Hospital to form Belle Point Hospital. Then the name of Belle Point was changed to Sparks.) Dr. Ludeau apparently moved away in 1917. [46]

Dr. Holt closed St. John's in 1934 and merged it with Sparks, where he became the manager. The vacant St. John's Hospital then became the home of Holt-Krock Clinic, and its patients were subsequently admitted to Sparks.

The other Fort Smith hospital, St. Edward (now Mercy Fort Smith), had its roots in the missionary activity of the Catholic Church in Ireland. Father Andrew Byrne, who had been born in Navan, Ireland, volunteered to come to the U.S. as a Catholic missionary in 1827. As a priest in New York City, he was ordained Bishop in 1844 and assigned to Little Rock, a diocese that included the Indian Territory as well as the state of Arkansas—but very few Catholics. One Catholic family had come to Fort Smith in 1840. Bishop Byrne, determined to establish a colony of Irish Catholics in Fort Smith, purchased a square mile (640 acres) of wilderness about a mile west of town that had been used by the U.S. Army as Camp Belknap. He borrowed the $5,250 purchase price from his brother-in-law in New York City. [47]

Camp Belknap was located on Section 16, and Immaculate Conception Church and its parish buildings are now situated in Section 16. The boundaries of Bishop Byrne's 640 acres are not specified, but they may simply have been the boundaries of Section 16. Inspection of a plat map of Fort Smith shows Section 16 of present-day Fort Smith to be bounded by Grand Avenue on the north, Towson Avenue on the west, Dodson Avenue on the south, and Greenwood Avenue on the east. With Bishop Byrne's audacious leap of faith, the Catholic Church now had more acres than parishioners in Fort Smith. General Zachary Taylor, the future president of the United States, was the commander of the troops at Camp Belknap. He and his troops fought in the Mexican War, and he returned from the war as the most popular man in the United States. When the war was over in 1848, Taylor was elected president of the United States. As for Camp Belknap, it was returned to the city of Fort Smith to be used as a site for public schools. The city then sold 640 acres of the site to Bishop Byrne to use the proceeds of the sale for building schools. "Despite a lawsuit filed by anti-Catholic factions in the Fort Smith area, the sale went through and the Church now had its first base in western Arkansas. Now it only remained to populate it." When a residence, thought at the time to be General Taylor's, was torn down, its chimney was left standing in its place and was converted into a grotto on the hospital grounds.

Needing Catholic pioneers, the bishop returned to Ireland and persuaded four Sisters of Mercy, with five postulants, to come back to "the wilds of Arkansas" with him. After establishing a ministry in Little Rock, the group of nuns split into two groups, and four nuns accompanied Bishop Byrne and his cousin to Fort Smith, where they arrived in January 1853. As they had done in Little Rock, they established a school—St. Anne's—as their first project.

The hospital came later. The sisters had experience taking care of the sick and wounded from both sides during the Civil War in Fort Smith, and some of these sisters were still living when they opened St. Edward's Infirmary (named after their Bishop Edward Fitzgerald) on November 27, 1905, after transforming their convent (built in 1876) into a hospital. Offices, six private rooms, and an operating room were on the first floor. More private rooms were on the second floor, and two wards—one for men and one for women—were on the third floor. A nursing school was opened in 1906, with four Sisters of Mercy among those in the first graduating class. Because the hospital had a waiting list for its thirty beds, ten more were added in 1907. One fourth of its patients were charity cases in the early years, and for nine years it was given an allowance by Sebastian County.

World War I delayed several building projects in Fort Smith, and among these was the new St. Edward's hospital on Rogers Avenue (then called the Little Rock Road), completed in 1923 with three floors and one hundred beds. The old infirmary became a nurses' residence, and the name of the infirmary was changed to St. Edward's Mercy Hospital. A fourth floor for obstetrics—delivery in a hospital was not common in rural areas at that time—was added in 1929. A six-story annex, featuring air conditioning, was added in 1953. Air conditioning was a novel feature in a decade when people would go to a movie theater just to find an air-conditioned place.

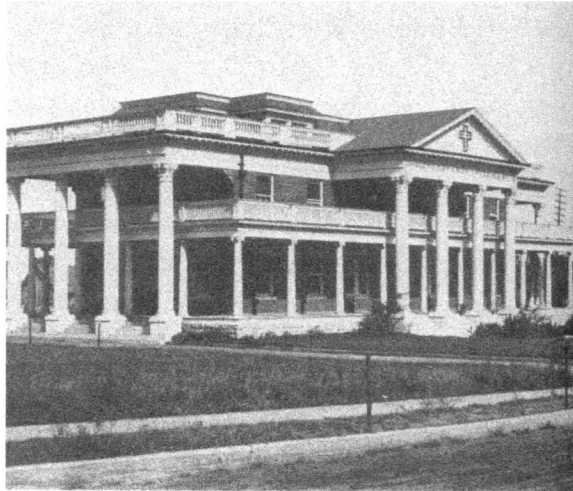

St. Edward's Infirmary was built in 1905, replacing a small infirmary that had been established on the same property at Fifteenth and Rogers in 1893. (Photo courtesy of Fort Smith Museum of History)

Baby Steps and Giant Steps in Patient Care

The Sebastian County Medical Society took its educational purposes seriously. Albert Dunlap, who had come to Fort Smith in 1852, presented a paper on cerebrospinal fever (meningitis) in 1874. Dr. James Edward Bennett, who had come to Fort Smith with the Union Army in 1861, reported that he had treated seven cases of cerebrospinal fever at the U.S. Army Hospital in 1863, with five deaths. Dr. Elias Duval, who later became president of the medical society in 1878, presented a paper on the changes in the treatment of pneumonia during the previous fifty years. Most members were reluctant to give up bloodletting, but Dr. Bennett reported that he had treated fifty-five cases of pneumonia at the U.S. Army Hospital in 1863, using no bloodletting, with success in fifty-two of the cases. [48]

Abdominal surgery, which had a mortality rate approaching one hundred percent before the advent of anesthesia and antiseptic techniques, was done with a fifty percent mortality in the 1880s and five percent mortality by the turn of the century. [49] A reason for surgery being done in the home, or in hotels or boarding houses, was the fear of infection that led hospitals to discourage their performance there.

The concept of antisepsis in surgery did not win immediate acceptance in America. Joseph Lister, professor of clinical surgery at the University of Edinburgh and renowned for his discovery of antisepsis, crossed the Atlantic to present his views to the International Medical Congress in Philadelphia in 1876. The response was mixed, some considering it a triumph, others reluctant to give up the concept of "laudable pus," without which they thought wounds could not properly heal. [50]

The importance of antisepsis filtered slowly through the United States and to Arkansas. Dr. J.W. Breedlove advocated antisepsis in the delivery of children in a presentation to the Sebastian County Medical Society in 1889; Dr. Earl Hardin agreed but doubted it would be feasible in his practice. Eleven years later Dr. D.M. Gardner reported his observations of aseptic surgery at Johns Hopkins Hospital, where William Halsted insisted on strict aseptic technique. [51]

The following was published in the *Journal of the Arkansas Medical Society* of April 1896:

> *We have boiled our hydrant water;*
> *We have sterilized the milk;*
> *We have strained the prowling microbe*
> *Through the finest kind of silk.*
> *We have bought and we've borrowed*
> *Every patent health device,*
> *And at last the doctors tell us,*
> *That we've got to boil our ice!* [52]

Infectious diseases continued to be a major problem in the early twentieth century. There were several fatal cases of diphtheria in 1910; tuberculosis was rampant in 1912; and malaria was a continuing problem. The First World War with its great influenza pandemic closed out the first hundred years of Fort Smith and its advances in medical care. Fourteen of the fifty-two members of the Sebastian County Medical Society served in the war. Surgery in Fort Smith was still occasionally done in the home, particularly for African-American patients who did not have ready access to hospital care. The house call was still a fixture in medical practice. Two clinics, Cooper Clinic and Holt-Krock Clinic, would be formed in 1920 and 1921. Sidewalks, drains, and sewers were in place, and new brick paving would be finally laid on Garrison Avenue in 1924. Though antibiotics were some two decades in the future, the public health measures were a powerful deterrent to the scourges and epidemics of the previous century.

Before proceeding to an account of the great influenza pandemic of 1918 and how it affected Arkansas in general and western Arkansas in particular, let us retreat to two small towns for the stories of two multigenerational families of physicians:

the Smith brothers of Paris, and their sons and grandson, and Dr. Addison Bourland of Van Buren and his son Dr. Othello Moreno Bourland.

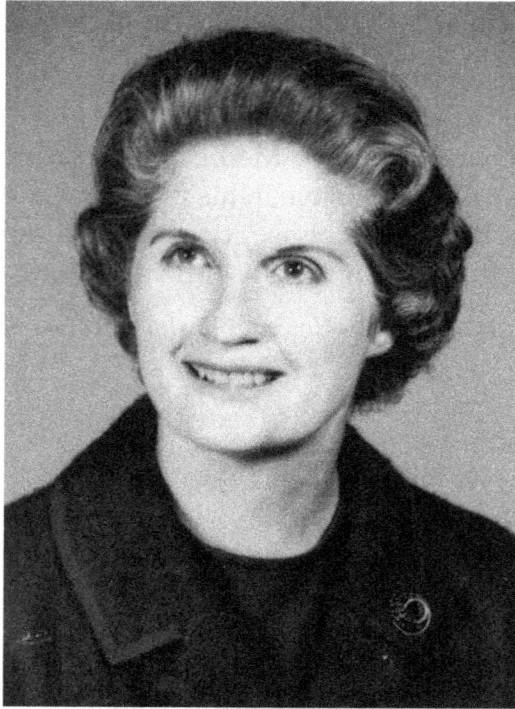

*Amelia Martin, wife of Dr. Art Martin, wrote **Physicians and Medicine: Crawford and Sebastian Counties 1817-1976**, an invaluable 647-page source of information. She was co-editor of the **Fort Smith Historical Society Journal** in 1977, the year the society was founded. (Photo from dust jacket [1])*

The Legendary Smiths and Their Paris Hospital

The Paris Hospital now stands empty. The Smith physicians who founded it and kept it alive until 1971 were remarkable men; local accounts of their accomplishments, particularly those of Dr. Jim Smith, the founder, and his nephew Dr. John sometimes push the bounds of credibility.

The First Generation: Dr. Jim and Dr. Mac

Arthur F. Smith homesteaded land near Chismville, Arkansas, in 1860, then died in 1863 in the Civil War. His oldest son J.J. (Dr. Jim) (1854–1941), attended a nearby one-room school and then taught school and took care of the farm to earn enough money to attend medical school at Vanderbilt University. He purchased what is now a long-deserted log cabin near Chismville for himself and his new wife in 1880, and there he established his practice of medicine. [1] Having taught his younger brother Arthur McDaniel Smith (1863–1930) (Dr. Mac), to read and write, he provided funds for him to attend medical school at Vanderbilt. When Dr. Mac returned and established his practice with his brother, Dr. Jim went to Jefferson Medical College in Philadelphia for further study. After Dr. Jim's return, Dr. Mac completed his medical studies at Tulane.

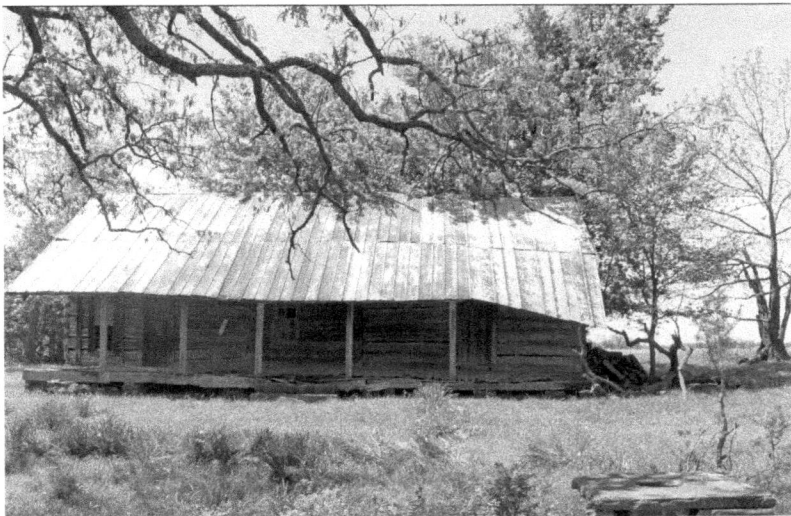

Jim Smith started his practice in this now abandoned log cabin near Chismville, Arkansas in 1880.
(Photo by the author)

Their widespread rural practice was the stuff of legend. They rode out in different directions each morning; a sheet hung out of a window told them which houses needed their services. Dr. Jim left his saddle and bridle on his fence so he could saddle up as fast as possible for night calls. He took a pistol with him on his rounds, using it once to shoot a pig when his brother Frank yelled at him to stop a pig that he couldn't catch. "Stopped it," Jim said as he holstered his pistol. [2]

They performed surgery within a fifty-mile radius from Charleston to Dardanelle. On more than one occasion they treated young boys kicked in the head by mules with elevation of the skull and insertion of a metal plate. One of these young lads survived into his seventies with the plate in place. They also performed laparotomies at least as early as 1900, draining an appendiceal abscess on one occasion and later removing the appendix. Surgery was usually performed on the kitchen table or under a shade tree, depending on the weather. They continued to occasionally perform surgery in the home through the 1920s. Dr. Jim performed much of the surgery until his late seventies when he assisted his brother. Dr. Mac, taller and quieter than his older brother, had a more calm and deliberate manner; yet the nurses stood in awe of him.

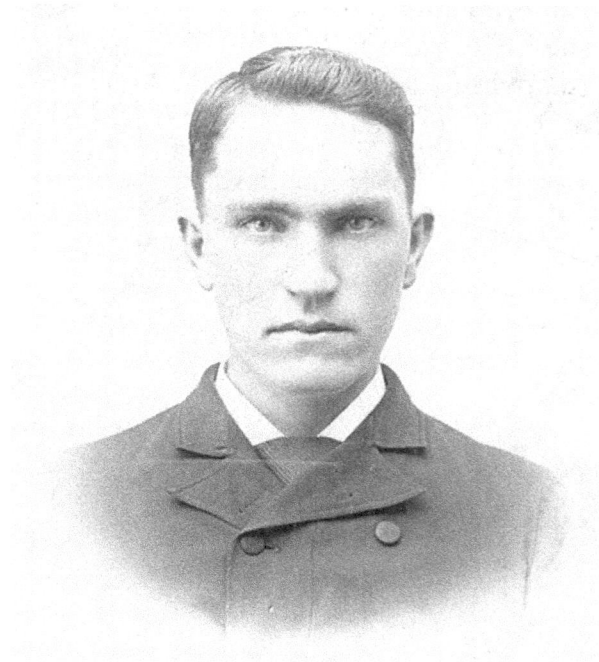

Mac Smith (1863-1930) was the younger brother of the first Smith physician Dr. Jim Smith (1854-1941). (Photo courtesy of Dr. J.C. Smith)

Dr. Jim moved his practice from Chismville to Paris in 1899, and Dr. Mac joined him in 1901. They opened a hospital in 1910 in the old Potts home and then completed construction of a new hospital on a hill in 1913, having to pump water up the hill from Dr. Mac's house. A three-story annex was added to the hospital in 1923, equipped with a three-story elevator and increasing the hospital's capacity to thirty rooms. [3]

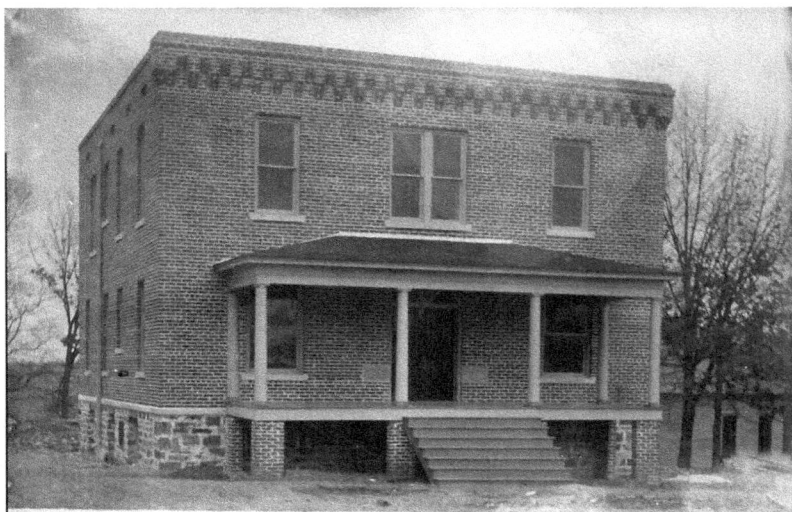

Dr. Jim and Dr. Mac finished construction on this two-story hospital in Paris in 1913. (Photo courtesy of Dr. J.C. Smith)

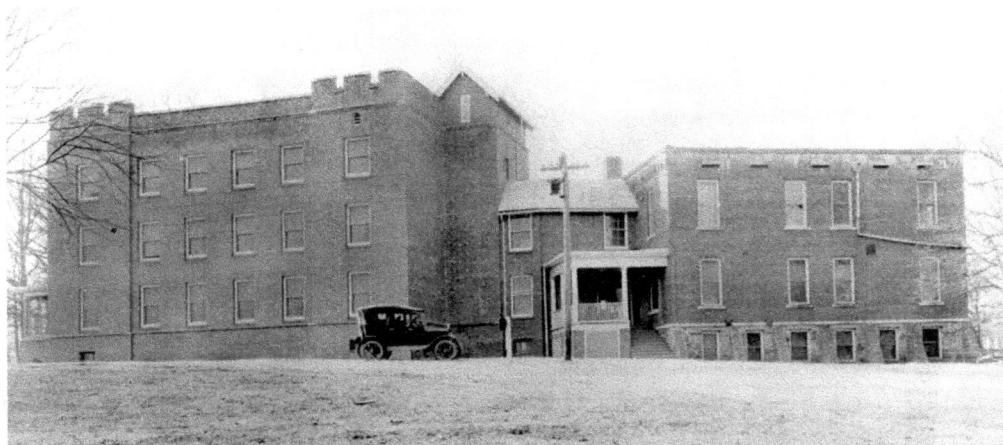

A three-story annex, shown on the left, was added to the original hospital in 1923. (Photo courtesy of Dr. J.C. Smith)

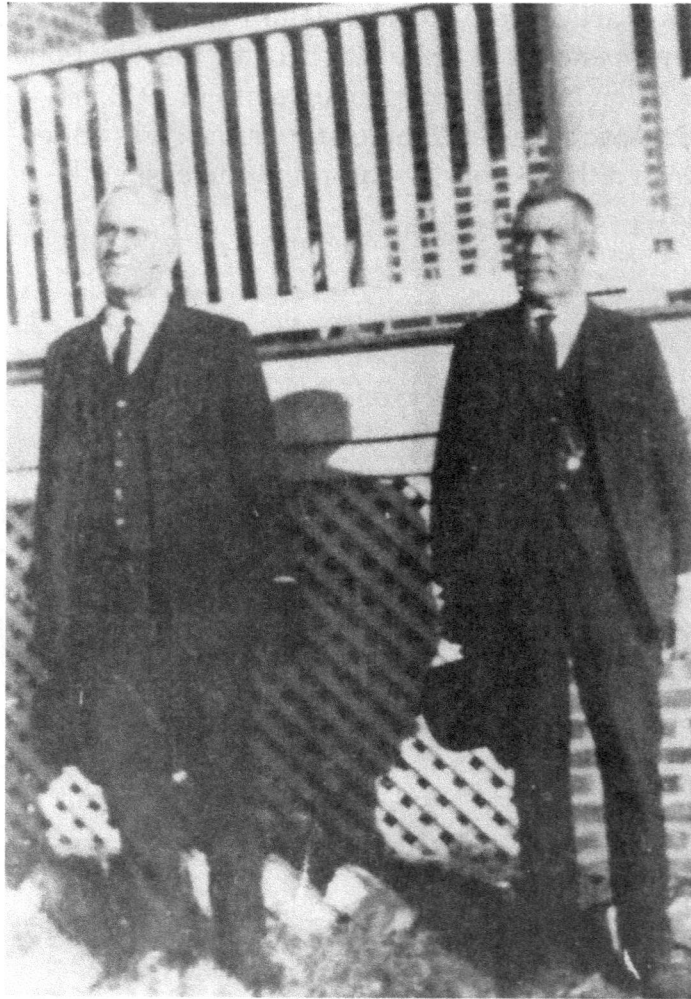

Jim Smith, on left, and Mac Smith, on the right, stand in front of the 1923 annex. (Photo courtesy of Dr. J.C. Smith)

"Any good surgeon," Dr. Mac maintained, "can also be a good mechanic," and family conversation at the dinner table often dealt with how things work: people's bodies, farm machinery, mining equipment, x-ray machines, pumps, corporations, automobiles. [4]

To provide affordable health care for the coal miners, the two brothers established a prepaid system called the People's Hospital Association in 1920, charging each family a dollar a month, extending the benefits and cost to two dollars a month in 1926. They also helped form the Fort Smith Colonial Hospital in 1928, operating on the same fee schedule of two dollars per family per month [5], later increased to three dollars a month with extra charges for a private room. They expanded the plan by offering it to the public. Though the American Medical Association did not object to prepaid medical care for specific groups such as miners, the AMA forbade provision of such a plan to the public. Dr. Jim relinquished his membership in the AMA. The Smiths sold their interest in the Colonial Hospital in 1930; it finally closed in 1952. (Holt-Krock Clinic began using the Colonial Hospital building in 1953.) [6] No patient was turned away from the Smith Hospital because they couldn't pay. The Smiths allowed the hospital to run at a loss, covering these losses with funds from other business interests. Though the mines closed, the public prepaid plan lasted until the hospital closed in 1971.

The Second Generation: Dr. John, Dr. Charles and Dr. James

Dr. Jim had no children, and all three doctors in the second generation were sons of Dr. Mac. Dr. John (1901–1960), the oldest, joined the clinic in 1925, Dr. Charles (1905–1979) in 1927, and Dr. Jim (1913–1994) in 1939. Dr. John became the administrator of the clinic. Having trained in pathology at Tulane, he had a basement dug for the hospital laboratory and personally directed its operations, sometimes staying until four a.m. to examine surgical specimens. Townspeople repeated many stories of his surgical prowess, some surely exaggerated. However, nurses affirmed numerous anecdotal accounts of his having reattached the chopped-off digits of farmers and miners. Operating on a victim of a stabbing, he found and sutured a laceration of the heart. Wiry and muscular, he went down into the coal mines to rescue injured miners. On one occasion he climbed a 150-foot wall, in suit and tie, with hat and lamp, to reach an injured miner. His domestic life was neglected for his work; he customarily left home at four a.m. and didn't return until nine p.m. Sometimes he would go to the local movie theater for a nap, leaving a young friend to come get him if there should be a call.

"Wound tight," competitive, and possessed of surprising bodily strength, Dr. John once arm-wrestled a heart failure patient to persuade him to take digitalis. He was known to lift the end of a car off the ground just to prove he could do it. On occasion, he would drop in at a local machine shop and do a few repairs. When he bought the first car in town with an automatic transmission, he drove it to a local garage and took notes while Joe the mechanic took it apart piece by piece. With all the parts on the floor, he gave them a few kicks. "Let's see if we've got it now." [7]

On one occasion Dr. John's father Dr. Mac called his hand. While assisting his father in surgery, Dr. John's hemostat broke in his hand. Swearing at the nurse, he hurled the hemostat across the operating room. In the silence that followed, his father looked steadily at him. "Why, Son," he said softly. Years later John's brother Charles clucked when he heard the story. "I'll bet John felt properly spanked." [8]

Although John virtually lived at the hospital, ate his meals there, and had no social life, he did buy season tickets to the Razorback football games, going to the most interesting games and giving tickets for the others to his brothers. [9]

Dr. John was almost overwhelmed by the volume of the practice during World War II when his two brothers, Dr. Charles and Dr. James, served in the military. Use of his left hand to position patients for x-rays resulted in cancer that started in the hand and required amputation. He used a hook on his forearm for the last years of his life. When he became terminally ill, he drove himself to the hospital where he occupied the otherwise vacant third floor and stayed there until he died, never seeing his wife again.

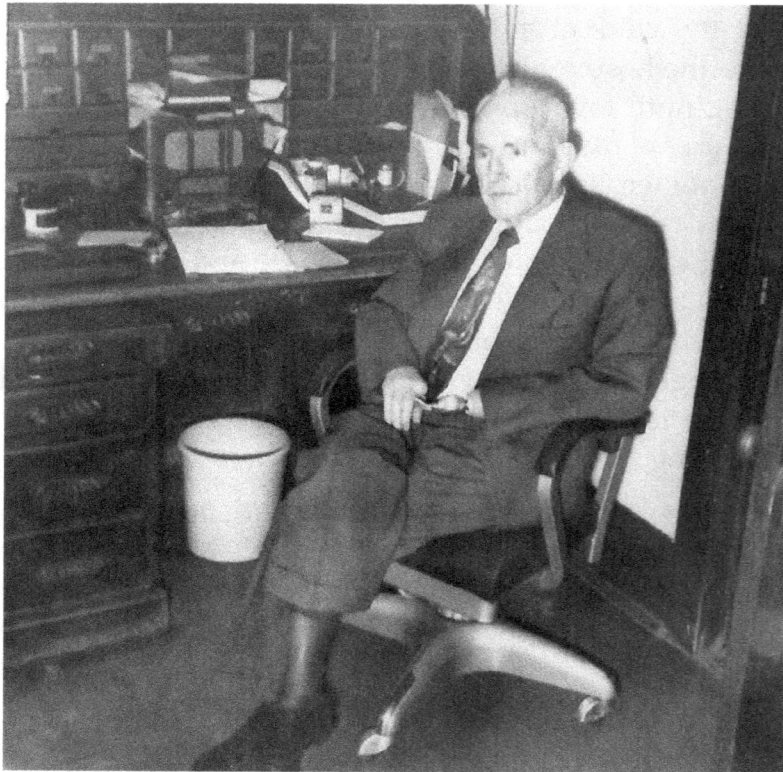

John Smith lost his left forearm to a cancer attributed to his practice of positioning patients for fluoroscopy with his left hand. (Photo courtesy of Dr. J.C. Smith)

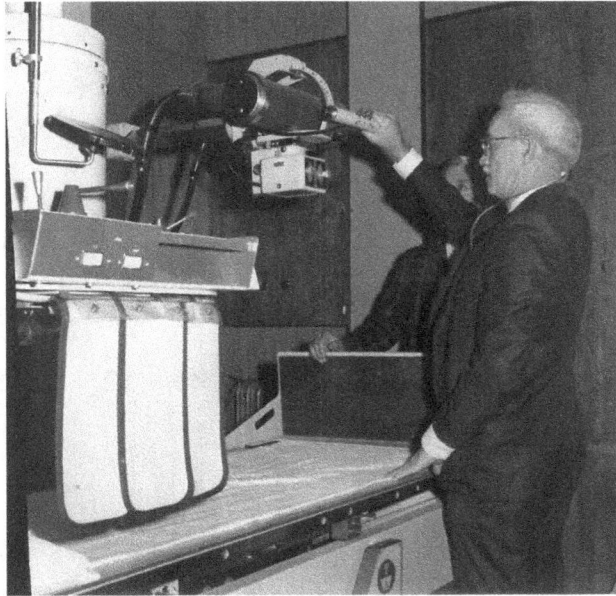

*James Smith shows an x-ray machine to the Logan County Medical Society.
(Photo courtesy of Dr. J.C. Smith)*

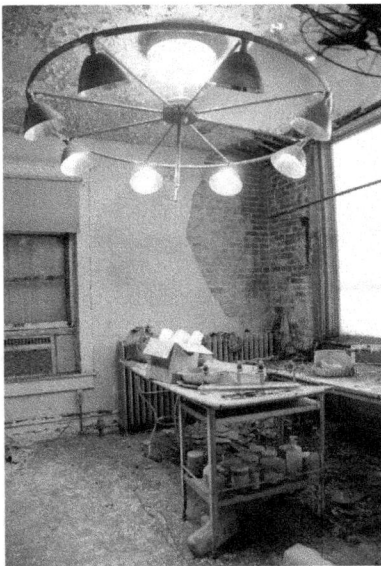

*The lights in the operating room still worked in
2013, just as they had when the hospital was
abandoned in 1971. (Photo courtesy of J.P. Bell)*

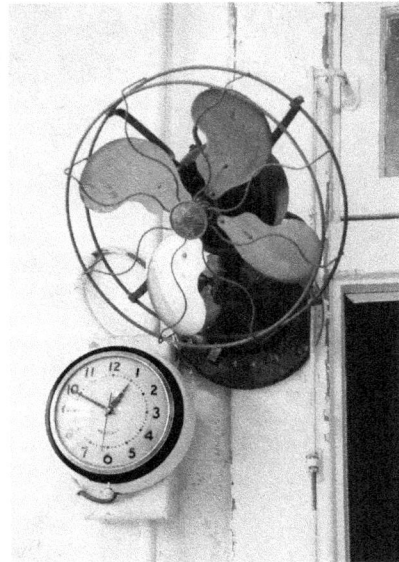

*The operating room was cooled by this oscillating
electric fan. (Photo courtesy of J.P. Bell)*

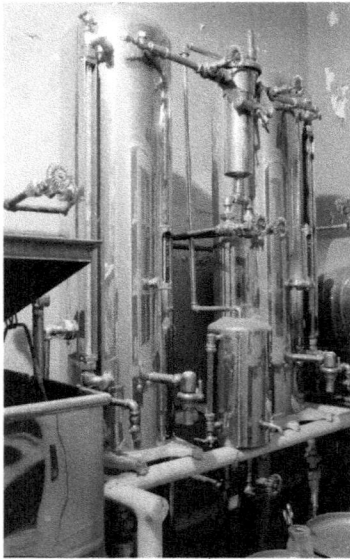

This steam autoclave was one of the reasons for the low infection rates. (Photo courtesy of J.P. Bell)

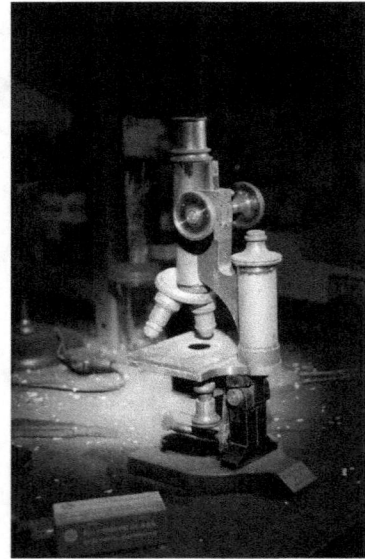

John Smith brought this microscope with him to start the laboratory in the basement of the hospital when he joined the clinic in 1925. (Photo courtesy of J. P. Bell)

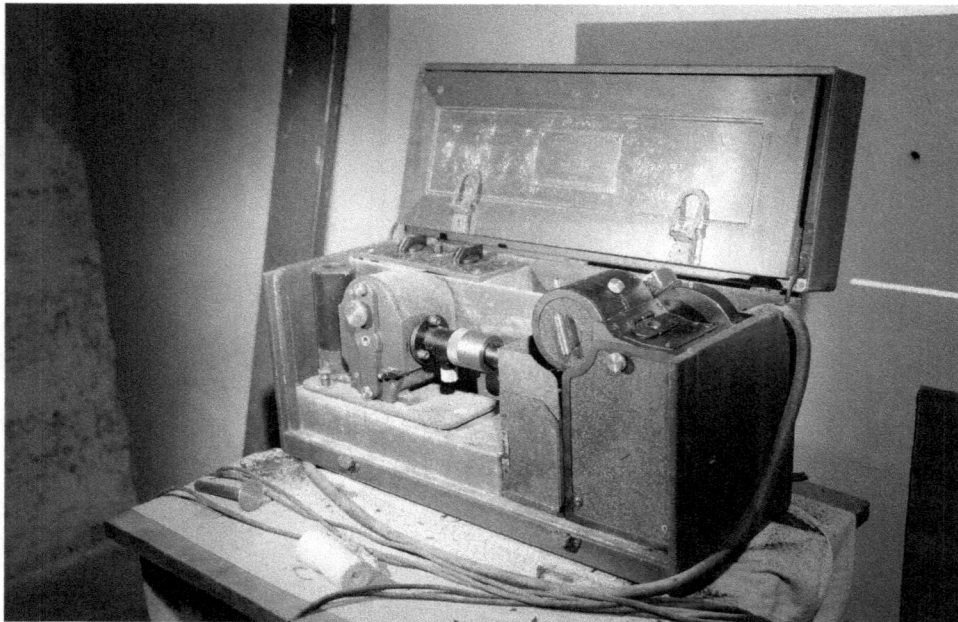

The brass plate attached to the wooden case of this EKG machine attests that it was made specially for the Paris Hospital by Cambridge Instruments. (Photo courtesy of J.P. Bell)

The hospital was an isolated institution unto itself. Dr. John found female companionship there. His brother, Dr. Charles married into the hospital in his own way. Geneva Campbell came to the hospital as a red-headed sixteen-year-old student nurse. Full of energy, she had many dates, none with Dr. Charles. Yet when she was twenty-two, and he thirty-two and father of two children, there was a divorce and he married her.

The hospital had loosened its rules for nurses by the time Geneva arrived. Until World War II nurses and students had to be single. They lived in the nurses' home and if they had dates, they had to be in by a certain hour. Young girls in their teens usually started work at this secular nunnery, where the head nurse was often called "Sister," with no previous health care experience or training. They took classes under the doctors and head nurses at night; during the day they received on-the-job training. Nurses did the janitorial and housekeeping jobs; they were paid thirty dollars a month, plus room, board, and laundry.

Some of the nurses became legends themselves. "As much a part of the hospital as the walls," Neecy Bradshaw was head nurse for many years, living first in the hospital, then in the nurses' residence, and finally in her own house south of the hospital, purchased with the help of the doctors. [10] She was the hospital anesthetist during the forties; after her retirement, all anesthesia was given by one of the doctors. Wilna Schnitzius Lawson (known as "Lawson") worked there until the hospital closed, as head nurse of the surgery unit and the doctors' office.

Dr. Mac died in 1930 at age sixty-six, Dr. Jim in 1941 at age eighty-seven, after retiring in 1936. Dr. James, youngest of the second generation, joined the clinic in 1939. A skilled observer, he once passed by Dr. John's examination room, looked in at the patient, and said, "Black widow spider bite." [11] Indeed it was, but Dr. James's own bite could be intimidating. Sometimes described as gruff and cantankerous, one patient said, "Aw, he barks some, but that's about all. He don't bite." Though he complained of the time consumed in obstetrics, Dr. James delivered 1,246 babies before his retirement in 1990.

With changes in economics and delivery of medical care, doctor-owned hospitals became a dying breed, and although the second generation of Smiths continued to subsidize the hospital personally, the brothers were obliged to close its doors in 1971. Dr. Charles and Dr. James continued to use the building as an office.

The Third Generation: Dr. John Charles

John Charles Smith (1948–), son of Dr. James, began work at the Smith Clinic in 1981, two years after the death of his Uncle Charles, who was killed in an automobile accident. John Charles had trained in surgery at the University of Oklahoma and was certified by the American Board of Surgery. He worked with his father until Dr. James retired in 1990; he continues to practice surgery in Paris and Ozark.

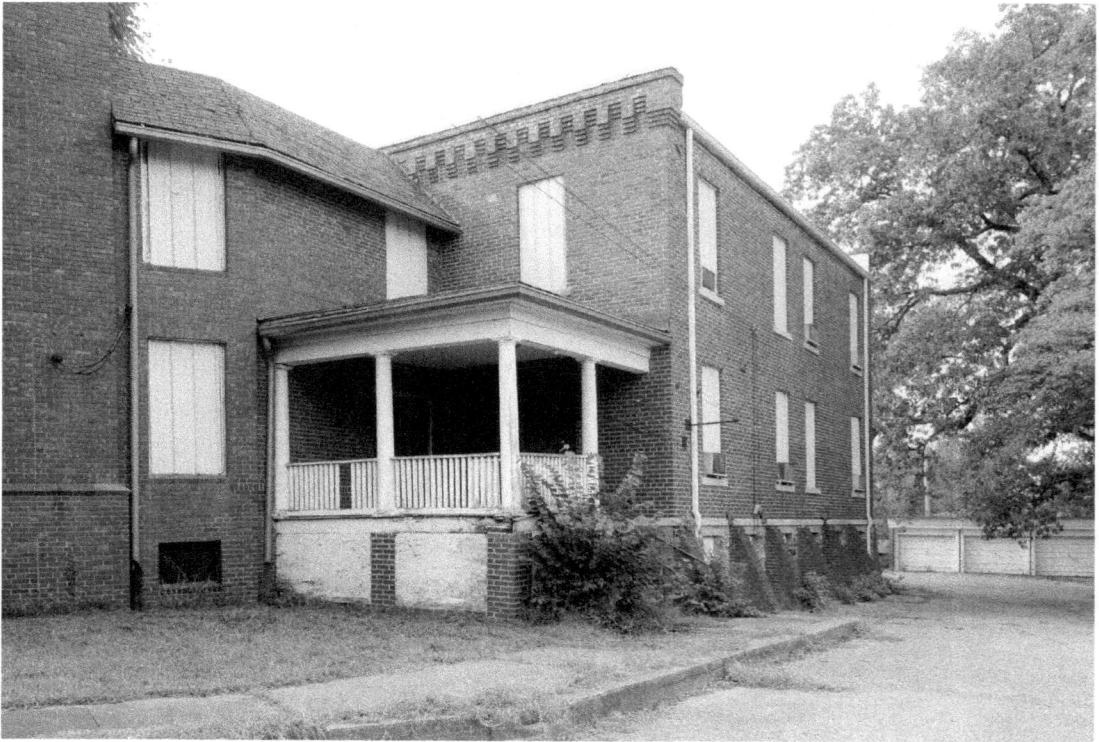

This 2013 photograph shows the abandoned hospital. (Photo courtesy of J.P. Bell)

The Doctor and the Mastodon

An Eccentric Naturalist, A Medical Practice and an Old Book

"Several weeks ago," *The New York Times* **reported** November 15, 1885, "the leg joints of some huge animal of the antediluvian period were found in the Arkansas Riverbed, about five miles above here." The dateline was Fort Smith, Arkansas. This "huge animal" was a mastodon, extinct some thirteen million years. "The cavity where the brain lay is perfect and indicates that the monster must have possessed more than a half bushel of brains." What happened to this find? "It will be sent to the New Orleans Exposition. The finders are searching for more of the skeleton." [1]

Though the "finders" are not named, one of the keepers of the jawbone of a mastodon was Dr. Addison M. Bourland, a polymath physician who collected and identified specimens from the streams and forests near his home. He added the "half under jaw" of a mastodon to his collection of fossils, which included various extinct ferns, trees, algae, and shells—and the largest collection of geologic specimens in the state at the time. [2] But a mastodon? Not quite so large as an elephant, the mastodon became extinct in the megafauna extinction that occurred shortly after the first delegations of *Homo sapiens* made their way southeast from the Bering Sea land bridge, probably about 13,000 years ago. Mastodons had already appeared some four million years ago and were stalking the Arkansas River Valley—in whatever form this Valley was—as the last glaciers retreated from their southernmost excursion to the Missouri River, about 11,700 years ago. Why did the mastodon become extinct? One theory is that changes in climate and habitat were the major reason. On the other hand, one can hardly ignore the coincidence of the disappearance of a large mammal with a low reproductive rate and a long gestation period, at about the same time as the arrival of a strange new species of two-legged hunter-gatherers from the Siberian land bridge. Indeed, sharp spear points have been found with some mastodon remains, and many of the skeletons show distinctive marks of butchering. [3] Here is a smoking gun that the jury is obliged to consider.

We do not really know when, where, or how Dr. Bourland acquired the lower jawbone of a mastodon. The Fort Smith *Elevator*, in reporting the finding of mastodon bones "on a sand bar in the river three miles below town" in 1890, alluded to a mastodon jawbone belonging to Dr. Bourland: "It has been now about fifteen years ago that a similar tooth, but smaller, and a section of the femur of some antediluvian animal were found on the same sand bar, and are now in Van Buren, in possession of Dr. Bourland. From time to time since then different fossils have been found, and a few years ago a number of large bones were found some six miles above here, but were evidently of a different animal from this one." [4] So Dr. Bourland's specimen may have come from a different finding. And for that matter, whatever became of it? And what happened to his collection of extinct fern and tree fossils? In a perfect world, they could be viewed in an Arkansas Museum of Natural History, or in a university museum, or in a local museum.

Not that there is a shortage of mastodon bones. It turns out that at least twenty mastodon skeletons have been found in Arkansas, more than in any other state in the midsouth region, according to the Arkansas State University Museum, which has a mastodon skeleton on display—found a few miles east of Jonesboro in 1999. [5] There is also a skeleton of an Arkansas mastodon in the Mid America Science Museum in Hot Springs. [6] And the remains of a mastodon were found on Island 35 of the Mississippi River in 1900, about four miles southeast of Wilson, Arkansas. The site has been destroyed, but a few fossilized bones are on display in the Hampson Archeological Museum State Park in Mississippi County, Arkansas. [7]

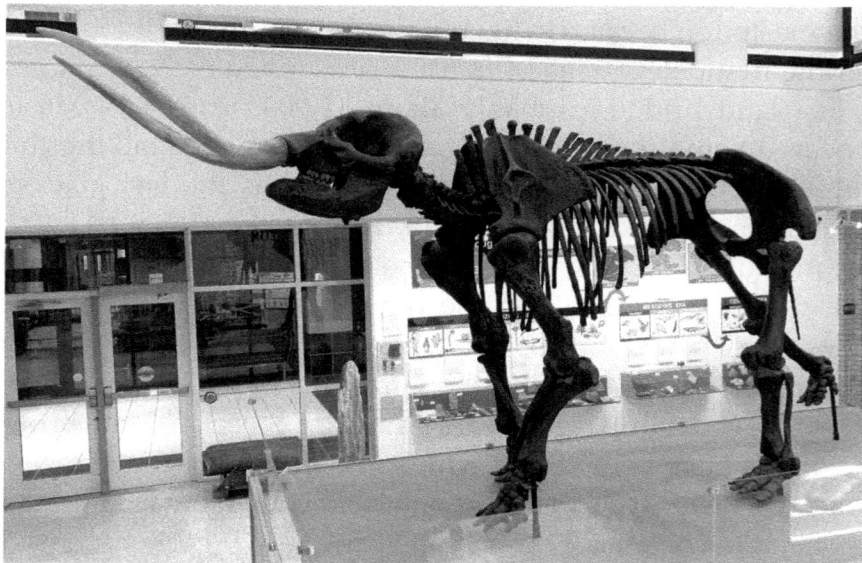

This mastodon replica in the Arkansas State University Museum in Jonesboro is composed of casts made from mastodon bones. (Photo by Sally Prewitt Maurras)

What does the lower jawbone of a mastodon look like? Three young boys in Mississippi found out when they came upon a strange object jutting out of the gravel on the family farm near Vicksburg in March 2018. It was indeed the lower jawbone of a mastodon, as identified by George Phillips, curator of paleontology at the Mississippi Museum of Natural Science. "I just saw it in the dirt," Caid Sellers said. "I thought it was a log, then I turned it over and saw the teeth. It was heavy. I tried to lift it. We all tried to lift it." [8]

Analysis of the teeth indicated that this mastodon was a mature individual, about thirty years old. Adult mastodons were eight to ten feet tall and weighed four to six tons, with tusks up to eight feet long, though not curved so dramatically as those of mammoths.

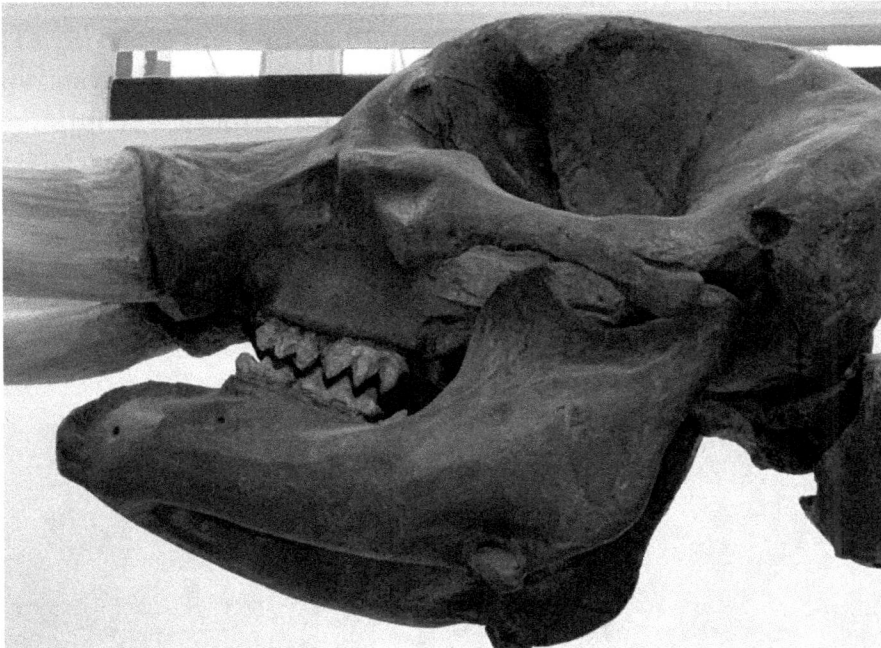

The tusks evolved from the mastodon's incisor teeth. (Photo by Sally Prewitt Maurras)

The first inkling of the existence of such a prehistoric "monster" came in 1705 in the Hudson River Valley in New York when the tooth of a mastodon was found in a field. [9] It was sent to Paris for identification; no one had ever seen anything like it. Was it from a race of giants? Was it from some terrible carnivorous predator? Analysis of the tooth indicated that it came from a herbivorous animal, not a bloodthirsty meat eater.

There was much speculation in the eighteenth century that this creature must have existed before Noah's flood, hence the term "antediluvian" [10] that persisted in *The New York Times* article of November 15, 1885, cited above.

It all became clearer when a nearly complete giant skeleton of a mastodon was discovered by some farmhands in Newburgh, New York. [11] Georges Cuvier of Paris gave this creature the name *mastodonte* (meaning "breast tooth" because the knobby points on the molars reminded him of nipples) in 1806, and now the American mastodon had a name.

Most of the mastodon fossils in Arkansas have been found along Crowley's Ridge or the Red River. But at least two and maybe three of them lived in the Arkansas River Valley and perhaps in the hills around what is now Fort Smith. Mammoths, more closely related to the elephant and even larger, have also been found in Arkansas, most notably the Hazen mammoth, found in 1965. [5] (The Hazen mammoth was not a wooly mammoth; the wooly mammoth was not quite so large, and its habitat was further north on the North American continent.) [5]

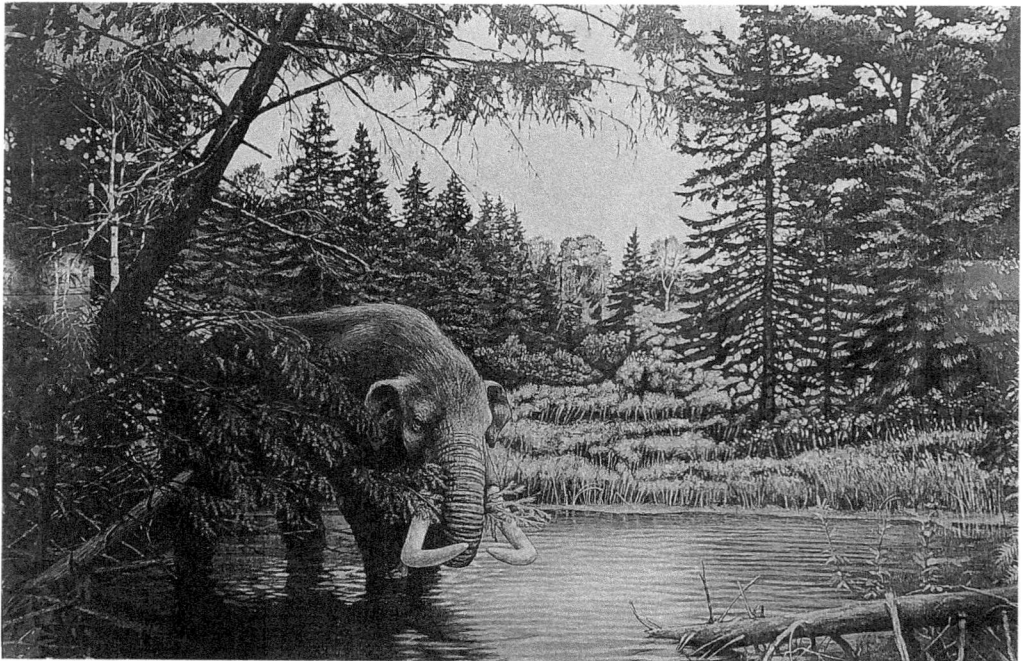

The mastodon stood about eight to ten feet tall and had tusks up to eight feet long. Illustration in Arkansas State University Museum (Photo by the author)

And who was this physician of many interests who collected and identified all these specimens from the streams and forests near his home? Addison McArthur Bourland practiced medicine in Van Buren from 1883 until his death in 1913. Amelia Martin's *Physicians and Medicine* [2] includes a photograph of him in the vigor of his later years—white beard, long white hair, and the wild-eyed look of a prophet.

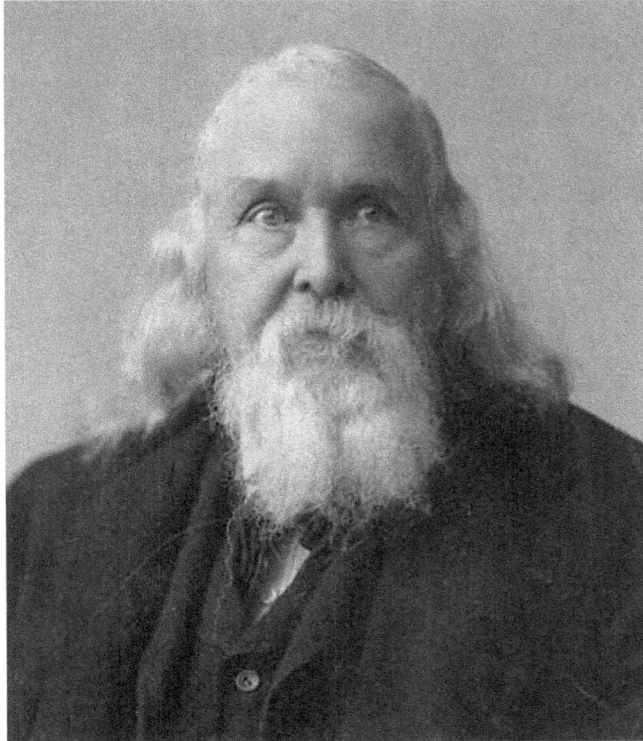

This portrait of A. M. Bourland shows the "eager, inquisitive countenance" mentioned in his biographical note in the Encyclopedia of the New West.(Photo from [2])

This prophet was no ordinary frontier physician. He was familiar with Latin, Greek, and French, and he had a French language medical library. He used the microscope in his private scientific investigations, taught school as a young man, home-schooled his children, and was a member of the American Association for the Advancement of Science. He became a charter member of the Arkansas Medical Society in 1875.

Not limiting his extracurricular interests to the field of science, Dr. Bourland wrote a philosophical romance, *Swanena*, describing the manifestations of religion in nature. He corresponded with the noted theologian J.E. Godbey, D.D., and he published their correspondence in a book, *Religion Philosophically Discussed*. [2]

Addison Bourland was born in Alabama in 1815 and, after his father's death, he began working on keelboats on the Mississippi River at age fifteen. He next studied medicine for two years under Dr. Barton B. Clements in Barry County, Missouri, before enlisting in the Arkansas Mounted Volunteer Cavalry to fight in the Mexican War in 1846, mostly serving as a hospital steward. After completing his one-year enlistment, he dispensed medicine in a United States hospital on the mouth of the Rio Grande. He moved to Franklin County, Arkansas, after the war, where he married Susan Davis in 1848. He saved enough money to study medicine at the University of Nashville, graduating in 1857 and returning to Franklin County to practice; his wife Susan died there in January 1859, one week after giving birth to their fourth child, Othello Moreno, who would later become a physician. [2,12]

When the Civil War broke out, Dr. Bourland served the Confederate army as senior brigade surgeon until the fall of Vicksburg. He participated in eleven engagements, serving as surgeon in all except at Dug Spring, where he fought as a soldier. He returned to Arkansas in 1864 because of ill health and began the practice of medicine in Van Buren. There he married Bettie Williams in 1865; they had two daughters, born in 1866 and 1877.

A serious unidentified illness in 1866 left him unable to read "without his whole nervous system being affected." [13] Although he could "see well," he required having someone to read to him. Despite this, he is described as being six feet tall, weighing two hundred twenty pounds, with blue eyes and "an eager, inquisitive countenance," with "great mental and physical strength, activity, and endurance."

Newspaper reports indicate that he retired from medicine after fifty years of practice, but a 1912 profile in the *Arkansas Gazette* stated that at age eighty-seven he would answer any call, night or day, summer or winter, two miles or ten, and that he had done more charity practice than anyone else in town. He was described as being a vigorous walker who had never used tobacco. He taught French and Greek classes in his home at no charge. [14]

He died "of old age" at age eighty-eight in his home in Van Buren across the street from the courthouse. There were conflicting reports of his health, the obituary stating that he had been a cripple for eight years, seldom leaving home, but "entertaining many callers on his lawn on pleasant days." [15]

Not mentioned in the 1912 and 1913 newspaper articles is the free spirit of his younger years. He organized the Secularist Society of Van Buren—"also known as Liberals, Agnostics, and the Society for Aesthetic and Ethical Culture"— upon his arrival in 1867 [16], later stating that he adopted no religious creed but inclined to the Liberal church.

The younger Dr. Bourland, Othello Moreno, grew up in Van Buren and attended Missouri Medical College in St. Louis, Vanderbilt University (graduating in 1881), and Bellevue Medical College in New York in 1883. [12] He practiced with his father in Van Buren for eight years, but they then dissolved their medical partnership and the son moved to a new office "uptown" in Van Buren while his father remained at the "old stand" at Second and Main Streets. [16] Dr. O.M. Bourland was third vice president of the Arkansas Medical Society in 1915; published scientific papers in the *Journal of the Arkansas Medical Society* in 1910, 1922, and 1930; and retired from medical practice in 1929 because of ill health. His wife was Ada Quaile Bourland of Ozark; he died in 1934, survived by two daughters and a son. [12]

It was the younger Dr. Bourland whose medical books had found their way, in 1973, to a small house on South Jenny Lind in Fort Smith where I spotted a "Books for Sale" sign and put on the brakes and turned in. I asked about one particular book that I saw.

"I'm selling these by the inch. This book is two and a half inches. That would be five dollars." I knew it was a rare book: *Principles and Practice of Medicine* by William Osler. On the inside front cover, in flowing cursive script, was a signature: "O.M. Bourland, December 1894." It was a first edition. There would be sixteen editions, but a quick internet search confirms that this one would be worth a bit more than five dollars—if it were for sale, which it is not. (I don't recall looking around the small house and noticing any strange rocks or fossils.)

And so, the Osler text sits on my living room bookshelf. Perhaps, in the next generation, it will not be sold by the inch.

When the Flu Hit Home

The Plague We Never Hear About

Fort Smith was shut down from October 8 until November 3, 1918, because of influenza. There were no church services or other public gatherings; no club meetings; no church weddings. All schools were closed. Pool halls were closed. Streetcars, normally crowded during rush hours, could only carry those who could find a seat. Public funerals were banned. (Funerals were to be private with only relatives and "immediate friends" present.) [1] The death toll from influenza was seventy-one in October 1918 [2] (total mortality that month was a record-breaking 119) [3]; but such numbers mean little. How many died after the quarantine ended November 2? What about Fort Smith citizens who died out of town? What about the numerous deaths of local men in the crowded army camps? There were some 7,000 influenza deaths in Arkansas in the great pandemic, more than triple the number in World War I, [4] but again no one really knows; rural deaths were often unreported. Influenza caused some 675,000 deaths in the United States, more than three times the number of American soldiers who lost their lives in the War—and more of these were due to disease (mostly influenza) than to combat. [5] Worldwide, influenza infected about one in four of the world's population. [6]

More than 115 deaths in one month in a city of about 28,000 [7]; as many as five were reported in a day--and yet this bit of history lies in a black hole of our collective awareness. It came and went so quickly, almost all in the month of October 1918. Few of the victims were prominent citizens; most deaths were among young adults in their twenties or early thirties. The war, nearing its victorious end, monopolized the front pages of the newspapers. And there was a curious mentality of keeping a stiff upper lip—stay positive so we can win the war, let's keep selling war bonds, don't risk demoralizing the folks at home.

There is no general agreement as to where the new variant of the influenza virus originated, but it appeared in American military camps in the spring of 1918. It struck a soldier at Camp Pike (later named Camp Robinson) near Little Rock on September 23. By that time 20,000 soldiers in camps all over the United States had fallen ill with influenza. Seven days later, there were 7,600 influenza patients at Camp Pike, of whom 100 died, in a camp numbering 52,000 recruits (making it the second largest city in Arkansas). [8] Troop trains spread the disease efficiently; of

3,108 healthy troops who boarded a train at Camp Grant in Illinois, "jammed into the cars with little room to move about, layered and stacked as tightly as if on a submarine as they moved deliberately across 950 miles of the country," over 700 men were taken directly to the base hospital on arrival at Camp Hancock in Georgia. The death toll from influenza was approximately ten percent of all the troops on the train. [9]

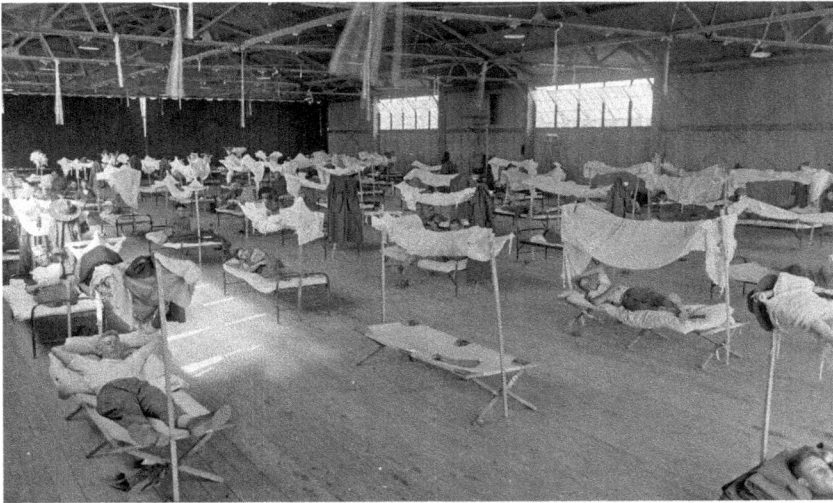

Overflow ward of Camp Eberts base hospital near Lonoke, September 1918
(arngmuseum.com /history/pandemic)

Statistics are not available for the number of Fort Smith men who succumbed to influenza in military service during the war. Eighteen deaths of men from Fort Smith and the surrounding area, or with Fort Smith connections, are mentioned in the *Southwest American* in September, October, and November of 1918.

The commandant at Camp Pike, "fearing panic as well as not wanting to appear unpatriotic in wartime . . . ordered that neither the extent of the epidemic nor the names of the dead be released to the press." [10] Dr. J.C. Geiger, U.S. Public Health Service officer for Arkansas, quoted in the *Arkansas Gazette* on September 20, called the threatening disease "simple, plain, old-fashioned la grippe" —a particularly bad chest cold. Even after quarantining whole families at Carlisle and confirming sixty cases in one day at Little Rock, Geiger acknowledged that the flu was worse than the usual grippe. But, he said, the situation in Little Rock was "not especially serious." [11] And after 506 cases of flu were reported in Little Rock and North Little Rock on October 4, with 296 cases more on the following day, Dr. Geiger reported, "Situation well in hand."

Before It Got Complicated

The state health department was preoccupied with promoting vaccination against typhoid at this time. [12] Only on October 4 were doctors notified that influenza was a reportable disease.

But this dog wouldn't stay under the bed. The story burst with sudden and unexpected ferocity. All of Camp Pike was placed under quarantine on October 3. Despite the quarantine, new recruits were pouring in daily. Little Rock was quickly swamped by the flu virus (nobody knew it was a virus; most assumed the disease was bacterial, attributing it to "Pfeiffer's Influenza Bacillus"). [13]

And yet the *Arkansas Gazette* reported on October 4, 1918, that the flu was beginning to go away. On the same day a humorous little poem about the flu appeared in the Fort Smith *Southwest American*:

THE LATEST WHEEZE
By Edmund Vance Cook

When your head is blazing, burning,
And your brain within is turning
Into buttermilk from churning,
it's the flu.
When your joints are creaking, cracking,
As if all the fiends were racking,
All the devils were attacking,
it's the flu.

CHORUS

It's the flu, flu, flu;
Which has you, you, you,
It has caught you and it's got you
And it sticks like glue.
It's the very latest fashion,
It's the doctor's pet and passion,
So sneeze a bit,
And wheeze a bit; —
           Ka-chew! chew! chew!

When your stomach grows uneasy,
Quaking, querulous, and queasy,
All dyspeptic and diseasy,
It's the flu.
When you have appendicitis,
Par-en-chy-ma-tous nephritis,

40

Laryngitis, or gastritis,
It's the flu.

When you have a corn, or pimple.
Complicated ill, or simple,
Broken bone, or fading dimple,
It's the flu.
When no matter what assails you,
If no doctor knows what ails you,
Then the answer never fails you,
It's the flu.

The Society column of the Fort Smith *Southwest American* announced rather flippantly under the headline "Until the Flu has Flown," "Those who were anticipating the pleasure of attending the war bridge at the Elks Club under the auspices of the Young Matrons Circle of the Patriotic League, YWCA, on Thursday afternoon, will have to curb their impatience, for the bridge has been indefinitely postponed until the threatened epidemic of Spanish influenza is over." (There were various theories as to why it was called "Spanish influenza"—it was unlikely to have originated in Spain, but since Spain was neutral in the Great War, its journalists were free of censors and could describe the disease in gory detail; and the King of Spain had the flu.)

It may or may not have been Spanish, but it wasn't funny. Four days after the light-hearted poem, on October 8, Dr. Charles W. Garrison, head of the Arkansas Board of Health, declared a statewide quarantine, closing schools and church services. The following proclamation appeared in the *Southwest American*: "In obedience to the instructions of the Board of Health all public assemblages are hereby prohibited within the limits of the city of Fort Smith from this date until further notice and all citizens are asked to lend their cooperation toward the enforcement of this regulation. The members of the grand jury now in assembly will be exempt from this ruling until their investigations have been completed. Arch Monro, Mayor—dated this eighth day of October 1918." [14]

This was on the same day that the flu epidemic made a rare appearance on the front page of the *Southwest American* (during October 1918 the war usually claimed all the ink on page one): "Physicians Must Report All Influenza Cases Now." However, the Fort Smith health officer said he did not think there was any necessity for closing of schools and other gathering places. In the following paragraph it was announced that all Van Buren schools were being closed, as well as "all shows and public congregations." This was immediately before Fort Smith was notified of the statewide quarantine.

At the same time the American Red Cross began to enroll nurses to fight the epidemic, and a call was made for volunteers to go into the homes where mothers and housekeepers were ill, and to "assume charge." [15] There were fewer nurses than doctors, and the Red Cross was not just "calling" for nurses. "(We are searching) from one end of the United States to the other to rout out every possible nurse from her hiding place." [16]

> Josey Brown was a nurse watching a movie in a St. Louis theater when the lights went out, the screen went blank, and a man appeared on stage announcing that anyone named Josey Brown should go to the ticket booth. There she found a telegram ordering her to the Great Lakes naval training station. [17]

Not that many nurses were available in Fort Smith, but there were volunteers, as described in this item in the *Southwest American*: "Mrs. Vick, who was one of the first to volunteer to assist the Red Cross in caring for influenza patients, has contracted the disease and is quite ill at her home North 18th and J Street."

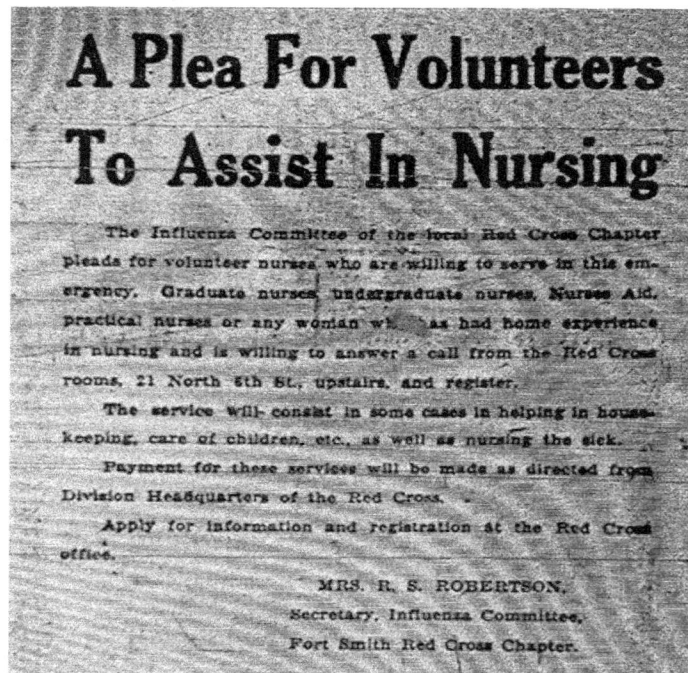

A Plea For Volunteers To Assist In Nursing

The Influenza Committee of the local Red Cross Chapter pleads for volunteer nurses who are willing to serve in this emergency. Graduate nurses, undergraduate nurses, Nurses Aid, practical nurses or any woman who has had home experience in nursing and is willing to answer a call from the Red Cross rooms, 21 North 6th St., upstairs, and register.

The service will consist in some cases in helping in housekeeping, care of children, etc., as well as nursing the sick.

Payment for these services will be made as directed from Division Headquarters of the Red Cross.

Apply for information and registration at the Red Cross office.

MRS. R. S. ROBERTSON,
Secretary, Influenza Committee,
Fort Smith Red Cross Chapter.

Those who volunteered to serve as nurses knew that they were putting themselves at mortal risk.
(Fort Smith Public Library)

One young Fort Smith man in the Navy had already died. The *Southwest American* had reported on September 25: ARCHIE BARTON DIES OF SPANISH "FLU" AT NAVY HOSPITAL. Young Barton had died in the naval base hospital in Philadelphia—" not quite fifteen years of age—he would have reached that age on November 19 next. He was a well-built robust lad, and he had no difficulty in getting into the Navy. He was the son of Mr. and Mrs. I.M. Barton of 1200 N. 8th St. He is a fireman on the Frisco . . . The lad's illness, it is believed here, was short."

Far too many of the cases, sadly, were all too short—sometimes leading to death after being perfectly healthy twelve hours before. [18] An Army physician wrote, "These men start with what appears to be an ordinary attack . . . of influenza, and when brought to the hospital they very rapidly develop the most vicious type of pneumonia that has ever been seen. Two hours after admission they have the mahogany spots over the cheekbones, and a few hours later you can begin to see the cyanosis extending from the ears and spreading all over the face, until it is hard to distinguish the colored men from the white . . . It is only a matter of a few hours then until death comes . . . It is horrible . . . We have lost an outrageous number of nurses and doctors and the little town of Ayer (Massachusetts) is a sight. It takes special trains to carry away the dead. For several days there were no coffins and the bodies piled up something fierce." [19]

Such was the case with David Brown, who died at age thirty-four. As described in the *Southwest American*; "The death was the most sudden recorded since the influenza epidemic reached this section. Brown was about his affairs Friday and taken sick that night with an attack of influenza which quickly developed into pneumonia complicated by a heart trouble," dying the next morning.

Charley Fountain, a twenty-eight-year-old conductor for the Frisco Railroad, was the first casualty reported in Fort Smith, survived by his widow and two daughters. He "died of pneumonia in a local hospital"; there was a reluctance to attribute deaths to flu if they could be attributed to pneumonia, considering this to be only a complication of influenza. [20]

Numbers were given in the reports from the health department reported in the *Southwest American*; the Society columns named names, especially in the Van Buren reports. On October 8, "It was reported yesterday that Dr. M.S. Dibrell was ill at his home. The physician had been called to Okmulgee twice last week to treat Dr. Herr of that city, whose case of influenza had developed into pneumonia. A message came yesterday from that city announcing that Dr. Herr had suffered a relapse and relatives in this city were asked to come." Dr. Herr died, thirty years of age, leaving a widow and two children, all of whom were also sick with the flu. He had practiced in Okmulgee for six years.

On the following day it was reported that Horace Hill and Will Kerwin, both attending the officers' training camp at Camp Gordon, Atlanta, Georgia, had been stricken with Spanish influenza and occupied adjoining cots in the base hospital.

By October 15—one week after the quarantine was ordered—the health department reported nineteen deaths due to influenza in Fort Smith, with 941 cases from October 8 to October 15, and forty-six new cases on the previous day. "There is a marked decrease and health officials feel the epidemic is on the wane." [21] However, two days later a headline read, "5 DEATHS AT FT. SMITH: Is Largest One-Day Toll Since Influenza Epidemic Began." [22]

Daily newspapers provide the closest approximation to a reconstruction of the number of cases and fatalities. The Sebastian County Health Department and the Arkansas State Health Departments do not have these records. [23] Kelly Scott described this phenomenon in his 1988 review in the *Arkansas Historical Quarterly*:

> A Rogers, Arkansas, journalist, Erwin Funk, accurately described the country's mood while on a trip to Chicago in October 1918. After relating how difficult it would be to gauge the impact of the flu in such a large city, Funk added: "Chicago is not doing any statistical gathering on the subject just now, at least for publication. Chicago isn't interested in the flu anyhow. Chicago is interested in the war." The same could be said about citizens of Little Rock, Fort Smith, or a dozen other Arkansas cities in the fall of 1918. The impending conclusion of the most catastrophic war yet endured by man proved to be an all-consuming topic for most people at the time, regardless of conditions closer to home. [24]

Two days later a headline in the *Southwest American* read, "DEATH RATE LOW FROM DISEASE HERE": "Out of about 1,200 cases of influenza that have been reported in this city the past fortnight there have been reported only 28 deaths from pneumonia, much of which followed the influenza . . . The figures bear out the statement made earlier that in this climate the disease was hardly likely to be as deadly as it had been in the North Atlantic states." [25]

Meanwhile, the society pages and the short news items continued their roll call. The words speak for themselves:

> The *Southwest American*, October 9: Dr. W.R. Brooksher is in Nashville, Tennessee, where he was called by the illness of his daughter, Miss Lucille Brooksher, who is suffering from an attack of pneumonia.

The *Arkansas Gazette*, October 14: Coal Hill–The influenza situation here is improving, only about 500 cases remaining. The physicians are badly overtaxed. The school and theater have been closed.

The *Southwest American*, October 15: The first official record compiled was on the 9th with 414 cases and one death after that day. On the 10th there were 91 new cases and one death. 11th–136 new cases and three deaths, on the 12th–122 new cases and two deaths, and Sunday the 13th–145 new cases and two deaths. Up to Sunday night there had been reported 898 cases since the inception of the epidemic.

The *Southwest American*, October 9: Dr. Holt Working Again
Dr. Charles S. Holt, who was confined to his bed at St. John's hospital last week with an attack of influenza, has recovered and is at work again, which helps to relieve the strain on the small corps of physicians who have been endeavoring to give required attention to the large number of people afflicted here.

The *Arkansas Gazette*, October 16: There is a marked decrease and health officials feel the epidemic is on the wane. Today's deaths increase the total since October 4, the date of the first influenza death, to 19. Keith Dyer, aged 19, local high school graduate, died at the University of Arkansas, where he was attending the Student Army Training Corps. Hubert Levi, Oscar Perry, Ernest Schlaeffli, soldiers of the city, died at Camp Maybry, Texas, Camp Dodge, Iowa, and Camp Sherman, Ohio, respectively. Earl Shipley of Booneville died at Camp Humphrey, Virginia. John Oliver of Greenwood was officially advised that his son, Sherman, American Expeditionary Forces, had died in France from the disease. Mary Leake, age 20, an employee of the government munition factory at Nashville, also died of the malady. Ninety-one of the 238 employees of the Fort Smith Wagon Company were reported ill today.

The *Southwest American*, Oct. 12 Sallisaw, Okla.: Seven members of the Brown family of eight, were placed aboard a Missouri Pacific passenger train last night and sent to a Fort Smith hospital, suffering with influenza complications.

The *Arkansas Gazette*, October 20—Decreases in the number of new influenza cases in Fort Smith yesterday and today assured health authorities that the epidemic was waning fast. Twelve new cases yesterday and nine today was the report. The death rate, however, continues. Since Friday night there have been 10 fatalities, bringing the total since October 4 up to 37.

The *Southwest American*, October 23—City health department death records show that in the first 21 days of October there were 60 deaths in the city and 16 bodies shipped here for burial in local cemeteries. Of these deaths the records show that 15 of the 16 cases brought home for burial had been due to pneumonia resulting from influenza. It must be remembered, however, that 15 or more of the 45 were deaths at local hospitals of persons brought from surrounding towns for treatment. Thus, the total deaths up to Tuesday of Fort Smith from influenza approximated 30.

(But there were still 60 bodies.)

The *Arkansas Gazette* Fort Smith, October 23 –Eighty-four new cases of Spanish influenza were reported here today, a marked increase over the past several days, and 23 more than recorded yesterday. From indications, the epidemic is not abating. There were two deaths today, including C.S. Carson, ticket agent for the Kansas City Southern Railroad.

GIRL AT FORT SMITH COMMITS SUICIDE

This headline in the *Arkansas Democrat* on October 25 reported that Martha Ramage, twenty, daughter of Theo Ramage, Rural Route Four, Girard Kansas, shot herself to death at a hotel that day (firing "a bullet through her right temple into her brain," according to the *Southwest American*). Her girlfriend died from influenza pneumonia the day before, and her sweetheart, Sid Donovan, died at three o'clock that morning from the same illness. On September 19 the girl had made an unsuccessful attempt at suicide with poison.

Although the suicide victim had a history of a prior attempt before the pandemic began, this incident gives some indication of the emotional and psychological effect of this overwhelming plague, only hinted at in most news reports and best described in works of fiction such as *Pale Horse, Pale Rider*, a short novel by Katherine Anne Porter. The author almost died from a severe case of influenza; she was in a coma for a month, and when she recovered, she learned that her fiancé had died from his illness. When she was becoming ill, she and her boyfriend sang an old spiritual they both remembered: "Pale horse, pale rider, done taken my lover away . . ."

After a hundred years, we don't hear many family stories about the 1918 influenza and its impact, but there are many of them. One friend recently told me that his father was born in Fort Smith in 1903, and his younger sister caught the flu in 1918 and died in less than forty-eight hours. She was about four to six years old. [26]

The *Arkansas Gazette*, October 26, 1918, NO SERVICES SUNDAY
Fort Smith, October 25–the city health authorities today declined to permit church services next Sunday because of the influenza. They received a petition from ministers of the city asking that the quarantine regulations be modified to

permit services. 31 new cases here today reported as having developed yesterday. Similar number was reported yesterday for the day before.

The *Southwest American*, October 29: 112 NEW FLU CASES
The health department records show 112 new cases of influenza for Saturday and Sunday, with five deaths, two of which were Saturday and three Sunday. The reports indicate new cases largely of a much milder form than in the early stages of the epidemic. After a conference yesterday the health department announced that unless there is a change from the rapid cessation of the epidemic the quarantine will probably be declared off next Monday and the probability that the churches will be released next Sunday from its restrictions.

The *Arkansas Gazette* Friday, November 8, 1918, SUCCUMBS ABOARD TRAIN
Fort Smith, November 7—While aboard a train going to a Fort Smith Hospital, Edward T. Lee, aged 29, of Quinton, Oklahoma, died from influenza yesterday. Lee was in a baggage car. Another influenza patient occupied an adjoining cot.

Three doctors in Sebastian and Crawford Counties died during the epidemic—Clark Wood, J.S. Ozment, and Edgar Lee Lindsey. [27] Dr. Wood was unmarried and died at the age of forty-one. He had served as president of the Sebastian County Medical Society in 1913. Having played football for the University of Arkansas, he refereed football games after beginning his practice in Fort Smith. [28] The *Southwest American* reported on October 22, "Up to a week ago he had been in robust health and was among the lead of Fort Smith physicians who were driven day and night in combating the epidemic. Not until the latter part of the week was his case thought to be serious."

Dr. Ozment died in Sparks Hospital October 16, 1918, at the age of 51. He and his wife had three children; he served as president of the Sebastian County Medical Society in 1915 [29] and was serving a second term as county physician at the time of his death. "Dr. Ozment was among the first victims of the influenza, which soon developed into pneumonia, and for the past week his condition has been held to be critical," his obituary reported.

Dr. Lindsey died in one of the recurrent outbreaks of influenza on February 8, 1920, at the age of 34. He had practiced in Fort Smith from 1914 to 1920, and he had served as secretary of the Sebastian County Medical Society in 1915; he was survived by his wife, his son, his parents, and his sister. [30]

Special to the *Southwest American*. Ozark, Arkansas. Oct. 19–Dr. George D Warren, one of the best-known and most highly respected practitioners of this section, died about 8 o'clock tonight of pneumonia following an attack of influenza. He was 34 years of age and is survived by his widow and one child.

"Every man's death diminishes me," but one of the great losses to Fort Smith was the death of Ben Kimpel of influenza at age thirty-five. A native of Dermott in southeast Arkansas, he was a graduate of the University of Arkansas and the Columbia University Law School. After beginning his law practice in Fort Smith, he joined Harry P. Daily in forming the firm of Kimpel and Daily. He was active in community affairs, and as chairman of the United War Work Campaign for Sebastian County he was representing this group at a meeting in Little Rock, where he was thought to have contracted the flu. [31] Under a headline, "75 NEW CASES OF INFLUENZA ARE REPORTED," the *Southwest American* reported in its second paragraph, "Dr. Hynes stated last night that no reports had reached the board yesterday of critical complications in any new cases, during the day. The most critical case yesterday was that of Ben D. Kimpel, who was reported last night suffering with double pneumonia and his family and friends much concerned over his condition." The newspaper reported his death on October 9 and subsequently his funeral at his home in Fishback Place on October 10. "The funeral . . . was announced as private but many close friends joined the relatives in paying the last tribute to the widely known young attorney . . . Many hundreds of absent friends paid tribute of flowers, and it was declared that a greater wealth of floral tributes was received than at any funeral for years." The Presbyterian minister was unable to officiate, having influenza himself, so another pastor conducted the service. The list of active and honorary pallbearers reads like a who's who of old Fort Smith: Robert Dickens, A.Y. Berry, Harry P. Daily, E.F. Creekmore, Robert Meek, W.H. Rector of Little Rock, L.H. Southmayd of Van Buren, T.C. Price, R. Scott Robertson, W.L. Seaman, Rudolph Ney, Judge Frank A. Youmans, Frank A. Handlin, Joe Ward, and Harry K. Albers. There were "hundreds of messages of condolence."

An ironic footnote to the story appeared in the *Southwest American* a few days later. A Sebastian County deputy sheriff was sent to Little Rock to bring back a man who was driving a car "in the jitney business" that had been stolen from Ben Kimpel several weeks earlier. "The defendant however was in the grip of a severe case of influenza and the officer was forced to come without him."

And a final footnote: the headquarters of the English Department at the University of Arkansas is in Kimpel Hall, named for Ben Kimpel, Jr., legendary professor of English there from 1952 until his death in 1983. [32] Dr. Kimpel had been a secretary to the U.S. Delegation in Vienna after World War II, before returning to Harvard, where he had been an undergraduate and graduate student. After visiting his mother in Fort Smith, he decided to take a position at the University of Arkansas. I remember his saying, when I was an undergraduate in the English department, that the only woman he would have ever considered marrying was Jane Austen.

Things can get a bit disorganized in a pandemic. Claude Marhanna, a Fort Smith cook, died at age thirty-six in Nashville, Tennessee. However, a "grave blunder," according to the *Southwest American*, by a Nashville undertaker resulted in the wrong body being shipped to Fort Smith.

It must be remembered that at the time, in the middle of it, no one knew how long it would last or how it would all end. Victor Vaughan, Surgeon General of the U.S. Army verbalized the sense of terror that was not unreasonable: "If the epidemic continues its mathematical rate of acceleration, civilization could easily disappear from the face of the earth." [33]

Although people continued to get sick and die, the numbers began to decrease in the latter part of October; and the first voices calling for an end to the quarantine came from the preachers, whose church doors had been shut. The health commission turned down an appeal from the clerical association to allow church services on October 24. On November 1, however, the state health department declared that the statewide quarantine was over, though individual communities might need to continue quarantine measures on their own.

This news was buried on the lower left corner of page two of the *Southwest American*, but the merchants and the churches sponsored large announcements. "The Lid is Off" called for early Christmas shopping, with an image of Santa Claus. "Come to Fort Smith to do your Christmas shopping. Come this week if possible."

The merchants of Fort Smith proclaimed their eagerness to resume business as usual following the lifting of the flu quarantine. This whole page advertisement appeared the following day in the Southwest American. (Fort Smith Public Library)

The quarantine ended in November 1918, but the flu was not gone. It continued its work throughout the last months of 1918, which are generally considered to be the second wave of the pandemic. The first wave was in the spring of 1918 and a third wave was in the winter and early spring of 1919. In time the death rate began to fall, attributed to mutation of the virus back to its mean, and because people's immune systems adjusted. [34] The flu continued to raise its head for several years, finally dropping back to its usual pattern in the mid 1920s. The year 1920 saw either the second or third most deaths from influenza in the 20th Century. [35]

Those who survived an attack of influenza were not necessarily well. The poet Robert Frost, months after recovering from influenza, wrote, "What bones are they that rub together so unpleasantly in the middle of you in extreme emaciation . . . ? I don't know whether or not I'm strong enough to write a letter yet." [36]

We don't know how many more died after the newspaper stopped counting at 119, in a city of 28,000. Once the war was over and the quarantine was lifted, statistical reports from the health department ceased to appear in the newspapers; and the health department itself no longer has the records. Compared to Fort Smith, Little Rock, with a population of 58,000, reported 9,813 cases of influenza during October; there were 351 deaths. At Camp Pike, there were 6,364 cases of influenza among the 51,956 soldiers stationed there. Of these, 79 died. (It must be noted that the previous month of September resulted in an additional 7,006 sick soldiers with 105 fatalities.) Nearly one in four people in central Arkansas became ill with influenza during September and October. [37] It may be that the death toll in central Arkansas was higher than in Fort Smith because Little Rock had already been poleaxed by the epidemic from Camp Pike when the statewide quarantine was ordered; the influenza may not have had as much time to catch a foothold in Fort Smith when the statewide quarantine was called on October 8.

There was a lot of doctoring, and doctors were indeed hard working and even heroic. But they had nothing effective to alter the course of the disease. Nurses, also exposing themselves to infection, had a better opportunity to tilt the odds a bit in the patient's favor. Laudanum, calomel, quinine, Tanlac stomach tonic (iron, thiamine, niacin, and ten percent alcohol), even face masks proved ineffective. Swamp Fever and Chill Tonic was manufactured by Morris-Merton Drug in Fort Smith. Daily advertisements, some in the form of news articles, in the *Southwest American* ran for the duration of the epidemic. A Morris-Merton Drug Company sign is seen on a building across Rogers Avenue from the Fort Smith Museum of History. [38]

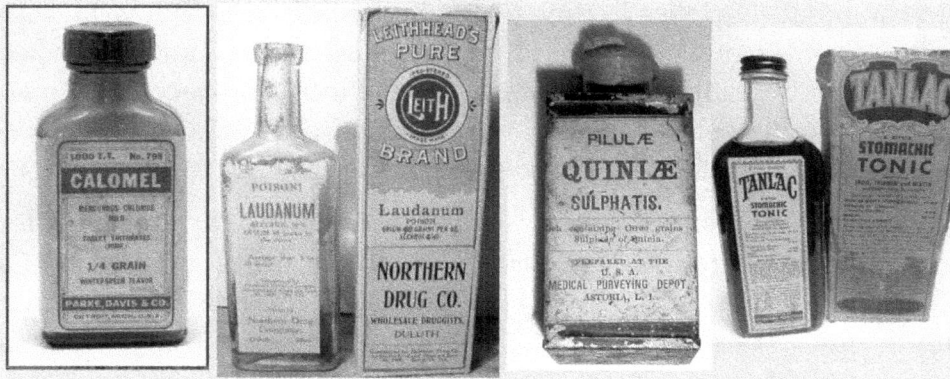

Nothing worked against the 1918 flu, but this did not discourage the pseudo-pharmaceutical industry. (Photo from Dr. Sam Taggart)

One thing did work; but it was in the realm of public health, not private practice: quarantine. The Arkansas State Tuberculosis Sanatorium in Booneville was placed under strict quarantine, closing its doors to everyone, and prohibiting all physical contact with the outside. There were no cases of influenza in the sanatorium. [39]

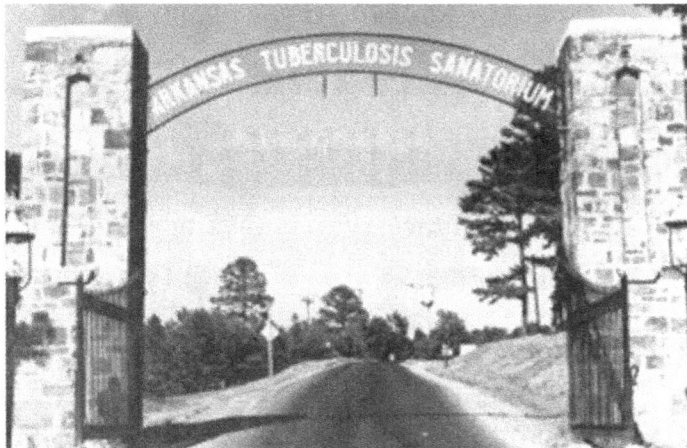

Arkansas State Tuberculosis Sanatorium had no cases of influenza in 1918 because of strict quarantine. (Photo by author)

Of course, this wasn't the last pandemic that the world will ever see. Will we be better prepared to deal with the next one? Probably not. The consensus is that the need for vaccines, medicines such as Tamiflu, hospital beds, ICU beds and ventilators would swamp the available resources. Ideally, a vaccine could be prepared for whatever new and lethal mutation of the virus may appear, but it will take significant improvement in vaccine preparation and production methods to provide adequate supplies in time to combat an infection that would spread so quickly in our interconnected world. It is hoped that a universal vaccine for influenza can be developed; but until such scientific and technologic advances appear, we would do well to remember one lesson from 1918: complete quarantine works—but you can't wait too long to get started.

For whatever reason, nobody talked much about the 1918 flu pandemic for a long time. Kim Allen Scott, in his review published in the *Arkansas Historical Quarterly* in 1988, attributed this comment to H.L. Mencken, the Baltimore journalist and (sometimes cynical) cultural critic:

> The epidemic is seldom mentioned, and most Americans have apparently forgotten it. This is not surprising. The human mind always tries to expunge the intolerable from memory, just as it tries to conceal it while current.

A few other major events of the time occupy this same black hole in our collective awareness. People in Tulsa are only now beginning to recognize what is now known as the Tulsa race massacre of 1921, which claimed some 100–130 African-American lives. [40] And in south Arkansas, nobody knew anything, until recent years, about the Elaine race massacre of 1919 that claimed the lives of an estimated 100–237 African-American lives. [41] I grew up in the area and may have heard a hint of it, but nothing was acknowledged. A friend of mine who grew up in Helena (twenty-five miles north of Elaine) in the 1940s told me a few years ago that she had never heard of it.

Influenza had nothing to do with race; who knows why such stories aren't told?

World War II had its own story that could not be told for decades: the Holocaust. It takes a few decades. It may take two or three generations. In the thick of battle soldiers keep their heads down and are too busy fighting to stop and reflect about it too much. When they come home, few of them are ready to sit down and give a blow-by-blow report of the fighting to those at home. That may come later—a lot later, usually.

Mankind cannot bear very much reality. It takes a while.

In the meantime, a few doctors in Fort Smith were deciding that things might be organized better. Two major clinics had their beginnings in the years just after the flu pandemic and the Great War, as we will see in the next two chapters.

Founding Fathers

St. Cloud Cooper, Charles Holt, Fred Krock and Their Innovative Clinics

For almost a hundred years, Fort Smith was the site of an innovative experiment in the delivery of health care—hardly original, but highly unusual, and unique in this area: two multi-specialty clinics, featuring division of labor to deliver medical care of the highest quality possible, in an era when the division of medical practice into specialties was still in its early stages. Cooper Clinic and Holt-Krock Clinics bore the names of their founders, emphasizing personal responsibility for the quality of care and establishing professional excellence as a high priority in a time when medicine was beginning to re-image itself from quacks and hucksters.

"An institution is the lengthened shadow of one man;" in this case, three men whose influence reached beyond their lifetimes, touching the lives of many who delivered and even more who received health care in this area.

St. Cloud Cooper

An old family story describes a young man, just off the train and looking around Fort Smith, when a member of the Gentlemen's Riding Club, sitting erect with whip in place and a robe across his lap in a buggy that was shined and polished, the horse prancing as if passing in review, turned from Thirteenth Street onto Garrison Avenue. The young man asked another onlooker who the driver was. Learning that it was Robert Meek (later to be owner of the Coca-Cola Bottling Company), St. Cloud Cooper said, "Well, I was just passing through Fort Smith, but if this town is good enough for him, then it's good enough for me." [1]

St. Cloud Cooper was born in 1861 in Jefferson, Texas. His father, Dr. John Cooper, served in the Confederate Army as a surgeon, and the family story is that Dr. Cooper, whose roots were in Carrolton, Missouri, was passing through Jefferson, Texas, in 1861 when he was pressed into service for the Confederacy. He stayed in Jefferson for the duration of the war, and then he rode his horse from Jefferson to Van Buren, Arkansas, where he was discharged from the Confederate service. He moved back to Carrolton, where his son St. Cloud attended school before attending medical school at Washington University in St. Louis, obtaining his MD in 1882. After practicing medicine in Tilden, Texas, St. Cloud Cooper did six months of post-graduate work in New York at Long Island College Hospital and New York Post-Graduate School. He then returned to his birthplace, Jefferson, Texas, and practiced there until 1895.

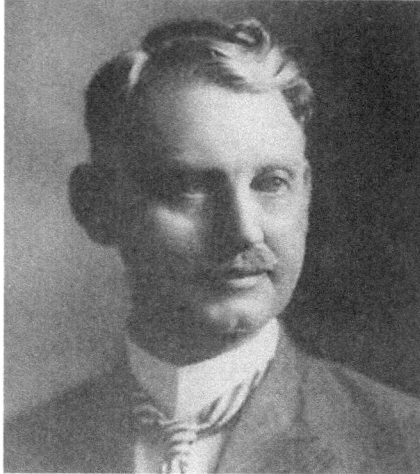

St. Cloud Cooper graduated from Washington University School of Medicine in 1882. (Photo courtesy of Joe Irwin)

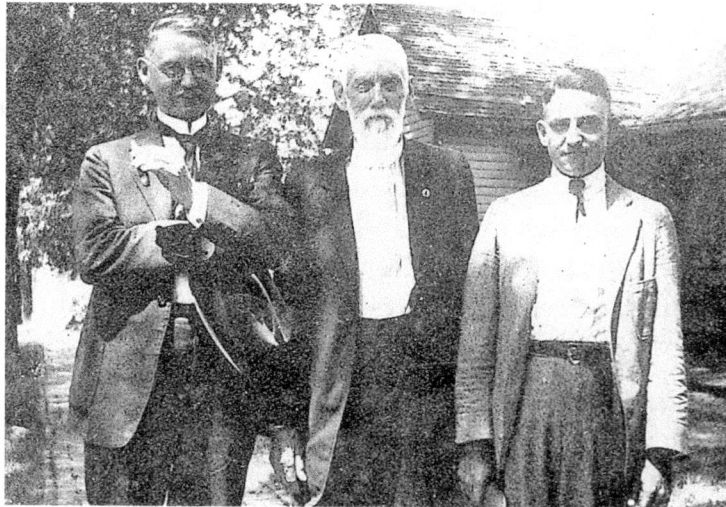

Hudson Cooper, son of St. Cloud Cooper, started a cattle ranch near Carrolton, Missouri, in about 1918. Dr. John Cooper, father of Dr. St. Cloud Cooper, lived in Carrolton and died in 1920. (Photo courtesy of Joe Irwin)

Dr. Cooper was thirty-four years old, and he and his wife Dora had three children—Charles Hudson, Lucy Kathryn, and Dora Bryant—when he had his legendary encounter with Robert Meek and moved his family to Fort Smith. Here he established his practice of medicine and became active in the Sebastian County Medical Society, where he presented papers on hypnotism, with illustrations, in 1901; successful treatment of tic douloureux by alcohol injections, with demonstration of injection of the gasserian ganglion; and gall stone and its surgery, in the early 1900s.

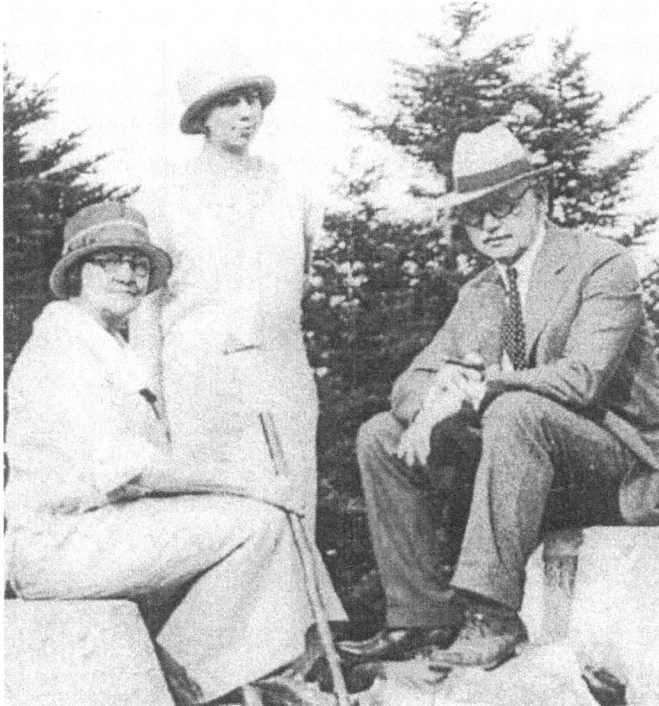

St. Cloud Cooper posed for this vacation photograph with his wife Dora and his daughter Kathryn.
(Photo courtesy of Joe Irwin)

Four years after beginning his practice in Fort Smith, Dr. Cooper served as president of the Sebastian County Medical Society, with a repeat term in 1909. He was president of the Arkansas State Medical Society in 1915 and president of the American Medical Association of the Southwest in 1916 and 1921. He considered his highest professional distinction to have been named a Fellow of the American College of Surgeons. He also served as president of the Fort Smith School Board and was a member of the Fort Smith Board of Health for fifteen years.

His idea of establishing a clinic maybe originated in the concept of "base hospitals during the war" and on the example of the Mayo Clinic, which had evolved from a partnership at the turn of the century and became known as the "Mayo Clinic" in 1914. Handwritten notes attributed to a reporter and dated September 26, 1920, state that the clinic would be conducted as a "group system." [2]

> The "group system" differs from the "cooperative group" chiefly in that it is more economical for the patients. In the "cooperative group" each member physician has his own executive force, makes his own fees and is in no wise responsible for the fee charged in consultation.

> On the other hand, a "group system" has but one executive office, one director, one bank account and the examination fee is made by the examining physician without regard or charge for consultation.

> . . . Dr. Cooper will be the directing head of the clinic, having conceived the idea for its organization weeks ago and selected the members of the associated staff.

> . . . Most of the members had experience in camps or in the war field during the war with Germany, became conversant with advances made in the preservation of health, surgery, and treatment of diseases during that period.

> . . . Hence of the two systems, the overhead expense to the patient is for the most part the examination plus the free consultation of all members of the group.

The "group system" is described as having evolved from general practitioners to specialists to the cooperative system to the group system, "such as in vogue at the Mayo Institute and as used by the army." "The clinic building is to be used for diagnostic uses only. The surgical work is to be done at St. Edwards Infirmary and Sparks Memorial Hospital."

(The concept of the free consultation, though never explained to me when I joined Cooper Clinic in 1969, appears to have persisted in the clinic culture until then but to have been time limited. I discovered that when I walked down the hall to ask a surgeon, dermatologist, or another internist for advice about a patient, they would immediately listen to my presentation, see the patient if necessary, and give me their recommendation on the spot. When I would consult a newer clinic colleague in this way years later, I discovered to my chagrin that the patient received a bill.)

The partnership agreement specified the following allocation of specialties:

> St. Cloud Cooper: consultant in surgery and internal medicine
> Miles Everett Foster: general surgery
> Sidney J. Wolferman: diagnosis and internal medicine
> Davis W. Goldstein: dermatology and radium therapy
> Holman B. Thompson: roentgenology
> Aubrey C. Belcher: urology and surgery
> William R. Klingensmith: internal medicine and clinical pathology

These allocations were not limiting; Dr. Wolferman did general and orthopedic surgery.

Dr. Cooper was director; Dr. Foster vice director; and Dr. Belcher secretary. Dr. Cooper was fifty-nine-years-old at the time he founded the clinic. The three others who remained in the clinic throughout their careers were significantly younger. Dr. Foster was thirty-three, Dr. Goldstein thirty-two, and Dr. Wolferman thirty-one. The three others were also in their thirties in 1920: Dr. Thompson was thirty-four, Dr. Klingensmith thirty-one, and Dr. Belcher thirty-one.

There is no evidence that billings and collections were considered in allocation of income among the partners, but income was not divided equally. The original interest of each of the partners was:

Dr. Cooper–28%
Dr. Foster–20.75%
Dr. Wolferman–15.75%
Dr. Goldstein–9.95%, decreasing to 5.75% for Dr. Klingensmith.

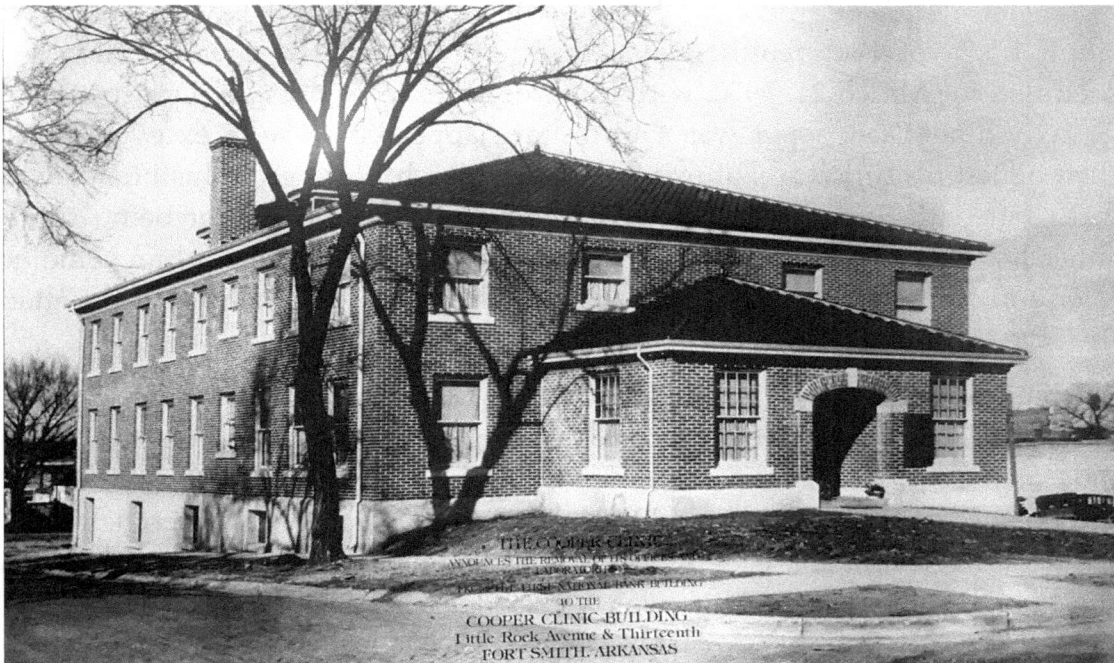

The message on this photograph, which was part of the historic exhibit in the Cooper Clinic lobby, announces the opening of the new Cooper Clinic Building on Little Rock Avenue (now Rogers Avenue) and South Thirteenth in 1924.

If clinic receipts exceeded a predetermined amount, the excess was allocated proportionately among Dr. Cooper's partners until their income matched his.

Dr. Belcher resigned in September 1921; Dr. Thompson resigned in 1924; and Dr. Klingensmith moved to Amarillo, Texas, in 1925. Cooper Clinic initially occupied the sixth floor of the First National Bank building on Garrison Avenue. Property for the new clinic building on Little Rock Avenue (now Rogers Avenue) and A Streets had already been purchased when the clinic was organized, and it was initially planned to begin construction within a few months. As it happened, the new building was built in 1923 and occupied in January 1924.

Cooper Clinic moved out of this building in 1972, moving to Waldron Road, and the building was subsequently used for the Area Health Education Clinic (AHEC), associated with the University of Arkansas for Medical Sciences, one of the first such clinics in Arkansas. After the building was torn down, it was used as the location of a sign for the adjacent bank, now the Cadence Bank.

Dr. Cooper published a paper on *placenta accreta*, said to occur once in about six thousand deliveries, in 1924, when he was sixty-five years old.

Joseph Irwin of Fort Smith relates that his birth by Caesarean section was scheduled for March 24, 1930, with the procedure to be done by Dr. Cooper. At age sixty-nine, Dr. Cooper was said to have appeared to be in excellent health when he left his office on Saturday evening, March 22, to go to his home at 104 North Fifteenth Street, only a few blocks away. [3] Shortly after being served dinner he told his wife he felt "indisposed" and asked her to get him some hot water and summon Dr. Wolferman; he was dead from an apparent heart attack when Dr. Wolferman arrived.

Dr. Foster performed the Caesarean section on Mrs. Irwin, and she named her son Joseph St. Cloud Irwin. Mr. Irwin was among the pall bearers. Joe says he has made many efforts to determine the reason for Dr. Cooper's name "St. Cloud," with no success. He has also tried to learn whether his parents and other family members called him "St. Cloud" or some nickname; but the only answer he has found to what people called him was "Dr. Cooper."

Dr. Cooper was buried in Forest Park Cemetery in Fort Smith. He was survived by his wife Dora, who died in 1950. His son Charles Hudson Cooper died in 1970, and his daughter Dora Cooper Beard died in 1986.

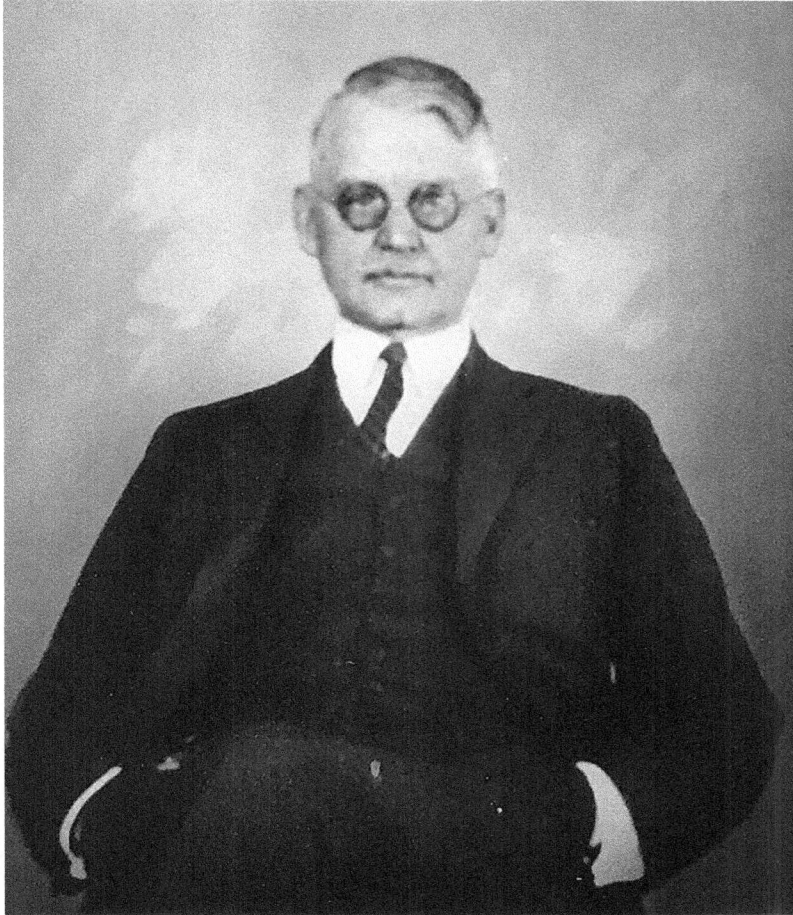

This is the most well-known portrait of Dr. Cooper; a copy of it, with his gold-headed cane, is a part of the historic exhibit in the lobby of the Cooper Clinic building, now Mercy Tower West.

Charles S. Holt

Charles S. Holt was born in 1880 in Salem, Illinois, to Thomas Jefferson Holt, a farmer, and Minerva Louise Holt. He received his MD degree at St. Louis University School of Medicine in 1906, interned for a year at St. Louis State Hospital, and opened his practice of medicine in the First National Bank building in Fort Smith in 1908. [4] He married Zoe (McCann) Bissell on September 30, 1909, and they had two adopted daughters: Betsy, who would marry Marvin Altman, long-time administrator of Sparks Hospital, and Zoe. [5]

59

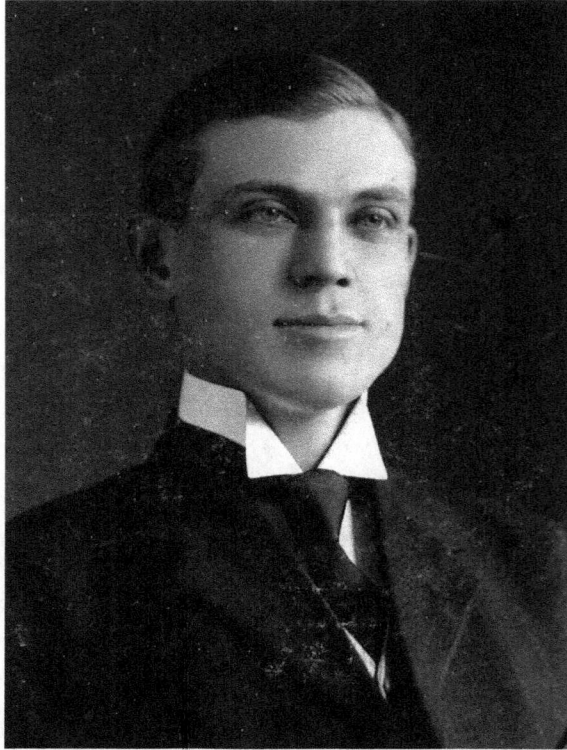

Charles Holt as a young man. (www.argenweb.net/sebastian/doctors)

Dr. Holt was a member of the city board of health in 1913, and for many years he was president of the board, involved in the passage of city food and health ordinances.

Dr. Holt and Dr. A.J. Morrisey bought the Ludeau Hospital, also known as the Fort Smith Hospital, in 1913; the new owners changed its name to St. John's Hospital. (As noted in the initial chapter, this made it a little complicated. The first private hospital in Fort Smith and in Arkansas is considered to have been St. John's Hospital, founded in 1887 by the Rev. George F. Degan, Rector of St. John's Episcopal Church. St. John's Hospital was merged with City Charity Hospital in 1899 and renamed Belle Point Hospital. Belle Point Hospital was renamed Sparks Memorial Hospital in 1908, and this is today's Baptist Health-Fort Smith, after a change of name and ownership in 2018.) Dr. Ludeau's hospital, with its new name of St. John's Hospital and probably located on North Eleventh Street, burned in 1914 and was rebuilt on 1425 North Eleventh Street, near the point where North

Tenth and North Eleventh merge to form Midland Boulevard. Dr. Holt bought out the interest of Dr. Morrisey and became the sole owner of St. John's Hospital. [6]

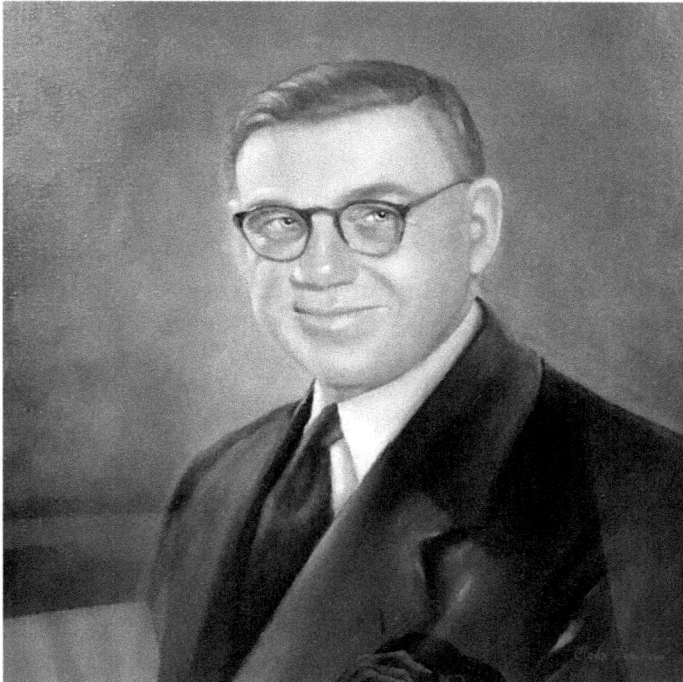

This portrait of Dr. Holt is included in the Holt-Krock archives at Baptist Medical Plaza.

A few years after buying St. John's Hospital, Dr. Holt formed Holt Clinic in 1921, with its offices on Texas Corner (Garrison and Towson), above the Fort Smith Drug Store. Charter staff members were:

Charles S. Holt– surgery and consultant
Leith H. Slocum– surgeon
H. C. Dorsey– diseases of the chest and medicine
Noble D. McCormack– diseases of infants and children
John Harvey– x-ray and pathology.

Dr. Holt found himself involved in a health care system far ahead of its time when he participated in the formation of the Arkansas–Oklahoma Industrial Hospital Association. Membership included all union laborers in the two states. and all members were entitled to receive free hospital or medical treatment at Holt Clinic or St. John's Hospital. Prepaid health care was anathema to the American Medical Association then, and the Sebastian County Medical Society filed charges against

Dr. Holt for unethical and unprofessional conduct. These charges were dropped when Dr. Holt declared that he would not participate in the association. [7]

Community activities included serving as vice president of the Fort Smith school board and, in 1923, as president of the Arkansas state school board. He was vice president of the Arkansas State Hospital Association 1930-1931; a trustee of the Arkansas tuberculosis sanatorium and of the Mid-West Hospital Association; president and director of the Peoples Loan and Investment Company; and a Fellow of the American College of Surgeons.

Dr. Holt was among those physicians who personally experienced the flu while making rounds on victims of the pandemic of 1918. Newspaper reports indicated that he was hospitalized at Sparks, and he did survive.

It was Dr. Holt who placed an ad in the *Journal of the American Medical Association* for a general surgeon, and in 1928 he received an inquiry about this position from a young graduate of Johns Hopkins School of Medicine who had stayed in Baltimore to complete a three-year residency in gynecology. His name was Fred Krock.

Fred H. Krock

Fred H. Krock was born in Upper Sandusky, Ohio, July 15, 1900, the son of Fred N. and Anna M. (Rock) Krock, and grandson of an immigrant who came to Ohio from Germany in 1843 and farmed four hundred acres near Upper Sandusky. Fred N. Krock took over the farm after his father's death, and his son Fred H. Krock helped on the farm, inventing a shut-off for the wind powered pumps that brought up the water for the cattle on the farm when the watering tank was properly filled.

For eight years the boy attended a one-room school to which the elementary teacher rode her horse from her home in Upper Sandusky. When weather did not permit travel on horseback, she spent the night with various farm families. Young Fred graduated from Upper Sandusky High School, then attended Western Reserve University in Cleveland, Ohio, because it did not have an ROTC program—his father was strongly opposed to military service.

The young undergraduate was inspired to go into medicine by contact with some fraternity brothers who were in pre-med, and by a botany professor who praised his drawings of plants. Fred N. Krock sold the family farm in 1919 and moved to Los Angeles, prompting his son to transfer to Leland Stanford University in Palo

Alto, California. There he received his BA degree and attended two years of medical school before transferring to Johns Hopkins in Baltimore where he graduated in the class of 1925. Medical specialties were in a formative stage in the 1920s, and Johns Hopkins was one of the centers where specialization was pushing ahead.

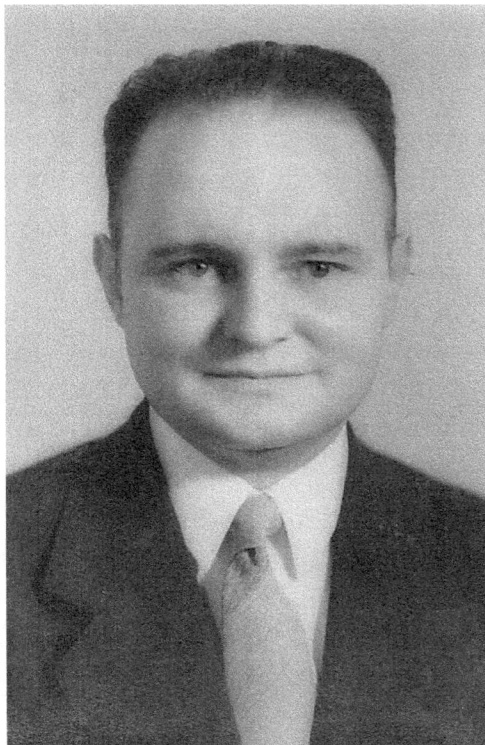

Fred Krock joined Holt Clinic in 1928 as a general surgeon after completing a three-year residency in gynecology at Baltimore Women's Hospital under Dr. Howard Kelly. (Photo courtesy of Dr. Curtis Krock)

The newly graduated Dr. Fred Krock completed a three-year residency at Baltimore Women's Hospital under Dr. Howard Kelly, who was one of the four founding professors at Johns Hopkins and has been credited with establishing gynecology as a specialty. During this time, he worked as an x-ray technician to earn extra money, but also learning to take films and develop them.

He had to obtain permission from his chief of service to marry; he married Hazel Armiger Josselyn in June 1927 at their summer house on the Severn River near Annapolis. They lived in his wife's parents' Baltimore home across the street from Johns Hopkins Hospital, except when he was on call at the hospital.

When he completed his residency in July 1928, the economy was beginning to falter even before the onset of the depression. There was an excess of gynecologists in Baltimore, but elsewhere his specialty was not so well established. He obtained a reference to visit a Dr. Wilson in Birmingham, Alabama, who told him he was having a hard time making ends meet himself and didn't need any help. Then he answered Dr. Holt's ad for a general surgeon. Though Dr. Krock was fully qualified in gynecology, he did not have formal training in general surgery. However, he accepted the position at Holt Clinic and became the fourth physician in the clinic, at a salary of $300 per month. (One of the staff members was a dentist.) He did his on-the-job training in general surgery by scrubbing with Dr. Holt, and he became a Fellow of the American College of Surgeons in 1933 and was certified by the American Board of Surgery in 1939.

While his wife was visiting her family in Baltimore in spring of 1929, he bought a home on 3700 Free Ferry (next door to Dr. Holt at 3620 Free Ferry). The philosophy of the Holt Clinic was to keep salaries relatively low so they could afford to add new doctors. Dr. Krock threatened to leave in 1933 because his salary had not been raised. In lieu of a raise, Dr. Holt reorganized the clinic as a partnership and changed the name to Holt-Krock Clinic.

Because of his moonlighting experience in Baltimore, Dr. Krock did the x-rays at the clinic and at St. John's Hospital. Since St. John's did not have x-ray equipment, he took the 150-pound apparatus to the hospital when x-rays were required. He then took them back to the clinic and developed the film, and if the x-rays had to be repeated, he hauled the machine back to the hospital again.

At first there was no pathologist, so Dr. Krock interpreted his own slides. He had had urology training in his gynecology residency, so he did urologic surgery. He set fractures and did other trauma care. He did emergency neurosurgical procedures, mostly burr holes for subdural hematomas.

Dr. J. Frank Blakemore related that when his wife came back ill from a foreign trip, Dr. Krock made a diagnosis of amebic dysentery; and when she was unable to stomach the pills he prescribed, he personally sugar-coated the pills to allow her to take them. He did one kitchen table operation when he did an emergency appendectomy on an eleven-year-old boy in his home in Mountainburg in 1931, using ether drip anesthesia. For this he was paid in twenty-dollar gold pieces. On another occasion he drove to a small town in Oklahoma to perform a subdural hematoma decompression. The patient recovered but was later sent to the state penitentiary for a felony.

Dr. Krock was a strong advocate for recruiting board certified specialists, and as new doctors came in, he was able to shed his duties in pathology, radiology, orthopedics, and neurosurgery.

St. John's Hospital merged with Sparks Hospital in 1934, and St. John's was closed. Dr. Holt became administrator of Sparks, and the Holt-Krock Clinic moved from its offices on Texas corner to the building vacated by St. John's Hospital on 1425 North Eleventh Street.

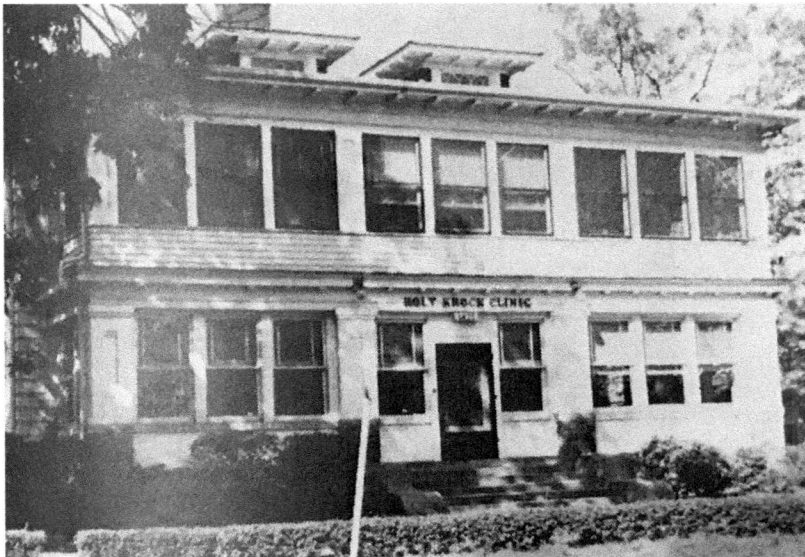

The Holt-Krock clinic after the clinic moved into the building formerly occupied by St. John's Hospital on 1425 North Eleventh Street in 1934. (Ref [9] of The First Hundred Years)

A banner headline on the front page of the *Southwest American* of April 3, 1934, announced: "DR. HOLT TO MANAGE SPARKS HOSPITAL." Dr. Holt's statement included: "When I realize that I am following in the footsteps of the eminent physicians who have been prominent in the management of the hospital in the past, it serves to emphasize to me what a task this will be. These men included Dr. St. Cloud Cooper, Dr. W.R. Brooksher Sr., Dr. Sam Brooksher, Dr. George Hynes, Dr. J.G. Eberle, Dr. B. Hatchett and Dr. H.C. King." [8]

Thinking that he could join other Arkansas doctors in a war he thought was coming, Dr. Krock joined the Naval Reserve in Arkansas in 1934. He was then ordered to active duty six days after Pearl Harbor—not with an Arkansas unit. He eventually became chief of surgery at a thousand-bed mobile hospital on Banika, a small island ten miles long and two and a half miles wide, west of Guadalcanal, being promoted to Captain by the time the war ended. After twenty-two months on this island, he didn't want to spend any more time on beaches or around palm trees, and it was many years before he agreed to take his wife to Hawaii. [9]

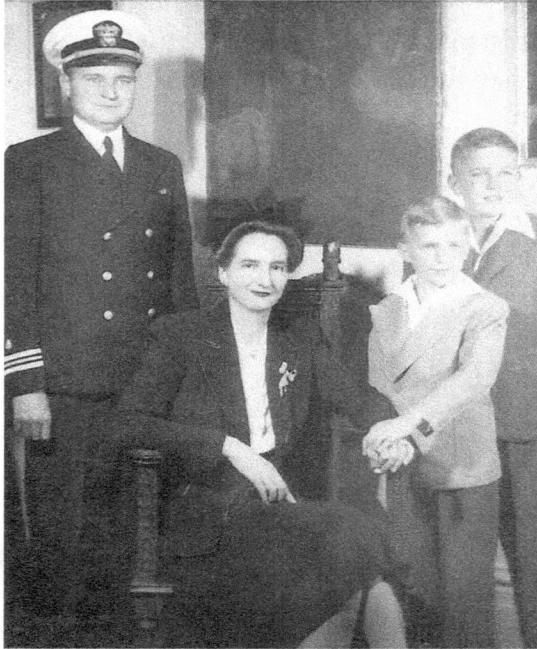

Fred Krock served overseas as an officer in the U.S. Navy during World War II. This photograph taken in Corpus Christi, Texas, in 1943 shows him with his wife Hazel and sons Curtis and Fred the eldest on the right. (Photo courtesy of Dr. Curtis Krock)

Dr. Krock served as president of the Sebastian County Medical Society, vice president of the Arkansas Medical Society, and was a Fellow of the Southern Surgical Association. He was co-founder of the Southwestern Surgical Congress and served as its president in 1961. Fourteen of his medical papers were published in various journals. (He was co-author with Dr. Sidney Wolferman of the Cooper Clinic and Dr. J.M. Taylor of a paper on arrhenoblastoma of the ovary published in *Surgery, Gynecology, and Obstetrics* in 1933.) He was also chairman of the Fort Smith American Red Cross, president of the Noon Civics Club, vice president of the Community Concert Association, and co-organizer and president of the Fort Smith Symphony Association.

His interests were wide-ranging. He learned to play the piano as a boy, and he later taught himself to play the cello. He sometimes played his baby grand piano at home before going to work in the mornings. His son Curtis played the violin, and when Dr. Krock saw an ad in *Popular Mechanics,* he ordered books about violins and began making them. (I heard his presentation about making violins at the Fort Smith Rotary Club, and I asked if he ever played the violins he made. He said he did not, but he did not mention that he played the cello and the piano.)

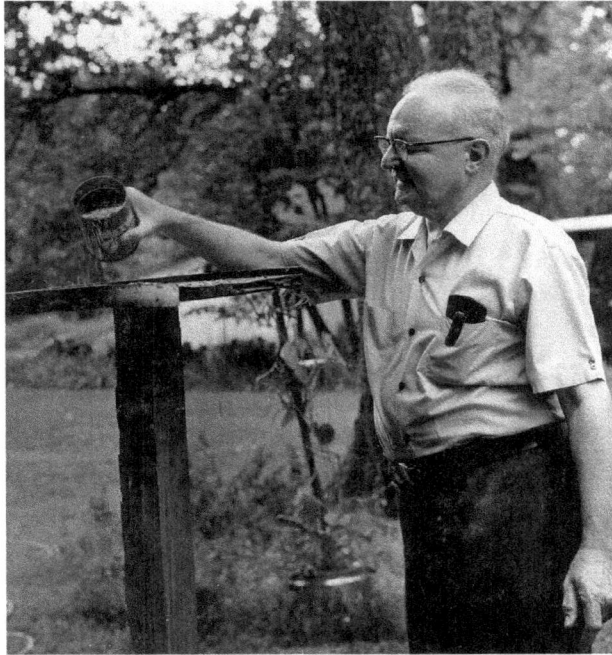

Fred Krock had many interests—among them, feeding the birds at his home on 3700 Free Ferry.
(Photo courtesy of Dr. Curtis Krock)

He ground a lens to build a six-inch reflector telescope; made a pair of golden candlesticks; made a grandfather clock that is now in Curtis's home; was interested in photography before the war; and obtained a short-wave radio and listened to broadcasts from South America and other parts of the world. He became interested in coin collecting after World War II and accumulated what was at one time the largest collection of ancient coins in Arkansas (mainly Greek and Roman). Curtis and his brother Fred now have hundreds of these coins. Curtis says that he enjoyed going on fishing trips with his dad to Lake Hamilton and other nearby lakes.

In the late 1950s he built an internal defibrillator for use in the operating room; he devised a boot type device that would alternately apply pressure and suction for the treatment of vascular insufficiency in a limb; and he made a nerve stimulator to help with nerve identification in the operating room during surgery.

Dr. Holt died of cancer of the prostate June 7, 1952, in Fort Smith; Dr. Krock died in May, 1981 of brain damage after a cardiac arrest.

Curtis Krock told me one last story. "One night one of the clinic physicians was called to come in to pronounce his patient dead. He declined coming in the night and said he would do it in the morning. The nurse then called my father who went in and pronounced the patient dead. The next morning, he called the physician into his office and told him that if this ever happened again, he would be fired immediately from the clinic."

The age of the clinics lasted almost a hundred years in Fort Smith. The names of the founders have been replaced by their successor institutions—the most recent Holt-Krock Clinic is now Baptist Health clinic on 1500 Dodson, and the most recent Cooper Clinic became Mercy Tower West on November 1, 2017. The delivery of health care has become more complex, and it's no longer so easy to know whom to call when a doctor fails to respond appropriately to a call in the night.

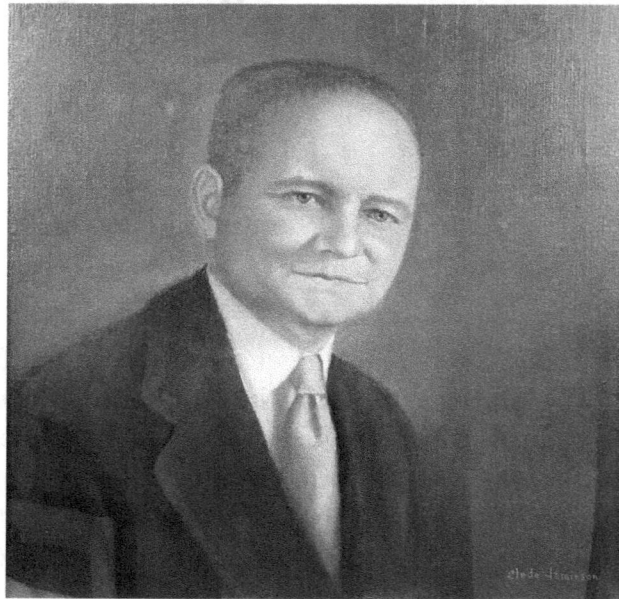

This painting of Dr. Krock hung alongside that of Dr. Holt in the Holt-Krock Clinic and is now in the archives at Baptist Medical Plaza.

There have been other heroes in the medical profession in Fort Smith, both within and outside the clinics that bore the names of their founders. But the names of St. Cloud Cooper and Charles Holt and Fred Krock meant something to the people in this area when they needed health care. The patient came first.

It's not so simple anymore, but the patient still comes first. Institutions have evolved and changed, but high standards continue. The shadows cast by these three giants of the past century have been long ones. Three of their successors joined St. Cloud Cooper in the founding of Cooper Clinic and represented the next generation of physicians. Fresh insight into how all this happened has just recently come to light in an exploration of—isn't it always a forgotten cardboard box? — boxes of original documents from a century ago. In the next chapter we'll see just what was in those boxes.

Present at the Creation

Miles Everett Foster, Sidney Wolferman and Davis Goldstein: Building a Clinic in Fort Smith a Century Ago

It was nearly a century ago that Fort Smith saw an innovative experiment in the delivery of health care when two groups of doctors left "private practice" to form two multispecialty clinics, Cooper Clinic in 1920 and Holt-Krock Clinic in 1921. [1] A valuable source of information about one of these clinics recently came to light as Cooper Clinic joined Mercy Clinic–Fort Smith on November 1, 2017, and donated its archives and scrapbooks to The Pebley Center for Arkansas Historical and Cultural Materials, located in the Boreham Library on the University of Arkansas-Fort Smith campus. Preserved in five cardboard boxes stored in a cabinet at the back of the clinic board room, historic documents were mixed with snapshots and newspaper clippings, providing a vivid picture of how medicine was practiced a hundred years ago.

Dr. Cooper was fifty-nine years old when he founded the clinic in 1920; the six others were in their early thirties. Three of these junior partners—Everett Foster, Sidney Wolferman, and Davis Goldstein—formed the backbone of the clinic and practiced in it for the rest of their lives. Another physician who would have a long and distinguished career, A.A. Blair, joined the clinic three years later.

This was a time when a doctor would stay up all night at the bedside of a child with acute appendicitis; a vacation to Colorado would be put off because a patient had typhoid fever; [2] the senior surgeon at Cooper Clinic would drive to Sallisaw to remove a gall bladder on the patient's kitchen table; and ham, eggs, and butter—on one occasion, a horse—were accepted as payment of fees without question. [3]

Miles Everett Foster

"I mashed my finger when I was a little boy," Irvin Sternberg recalls, "and when Dr. Foster was inspecting it, he saw that I was about to faint, and he had me hold my head down." This was the same gruff surgeon whom his office nurse Ann (Polla) Miller described as striking fear in the hearts of nurses and cursing under his breath (and perhaps merely more frequently and loudly than usual) when he had to operate on an overweight patient.

Miles Everett Foster, Sr., was born in Witcherville, Arkansas, January 4, 1887, to Dr. James H. and Christine Foster. He graduated from Fort Smith High School and was valedictorian of his class at Jefferson Medical School in Philadelphia in 1906. After an internship at Atlantic City Hospital in, New Jersey, he did a surgery residency at Jefferson Medical College Hospital in Philadelphia. He practiced with his father in Fort Smith from 1911 until he entered military service during World War I, at which time he was sent to Barnes Hospital in St. Louis for training in plastic surgery under Dr. Vilray Blair, commander of the U.S. Army Corps of Head and Neck Surgeons. Dr. Foster served as executive officer and chief of plastic surgery with the 42nd General Hospital Center. He received the European Theater Ribbon and the Croix de Guerre. [4]

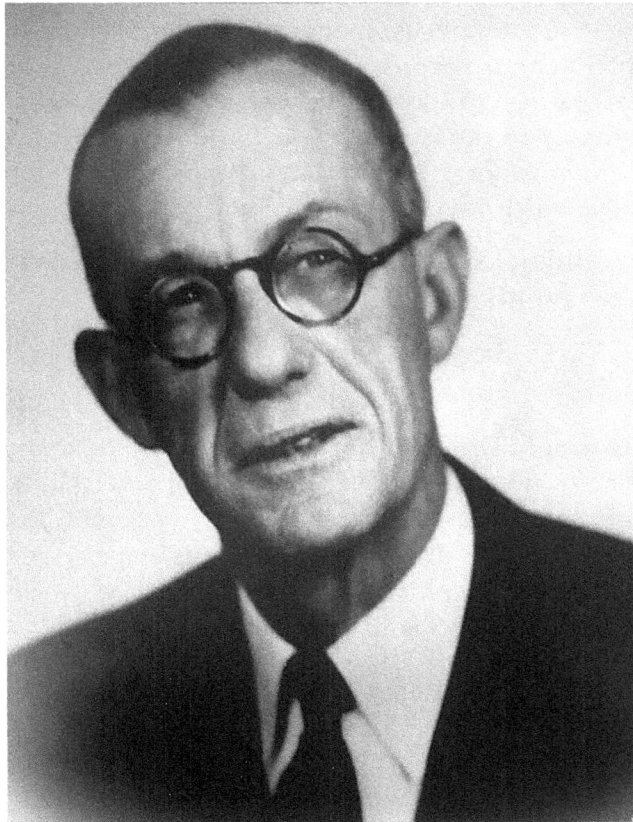

Portrait of Miles Everett Foster hanging in the old Cooper Clinic main lobby.

After the war he entered practice in Fort Smith and joined Dr. St. Cloud Cooper in planning the formation of Cooper Clinic, going with him and Dr. Sidney Wolferman to Rochester, Minnesota, to study the organization of the Mayo Clinic

71

as a model. Each partner's income was based on a predetermined percentage. Dr. Foster's job description was "General Surgery." [5]

Dr. Foster was a member of the American College of Surgeons and served as president of the Sebastian County Medical Society in 1936. He succeeded Dr. Cooper as president of Cooper Clinic and served many terms as chief of staff at St. Edward Mercy Hospital. He was a member of the First Presbyterian Church and Hardscrabble Country Club. [6]

A rather informal insight into Dr. Foster's clinical interests is found in a comment on a colleague's paper presented at the Arkansas State Medical Society meeting, recorded in the *Journal of the Arkansas Medical Society* in 1933:

> I was very much excited last week. I saw a woman, age sixty-five, with a small movable mass near the umbilicus, marked visible peristaltic waves, history of alternate constipation and diarrhea, no vomiting, a sensation of fullness, with pain at times after eating, and I thought we were going to add another case of small intestinal tumor to our series of one. The X-ray, however, spoiled our playhouse, as the roentgenologist gave us a diagnosis of carcinoma of the pyloric end of the stomach, which was verified several days later by operation. [7]

His plastic surgery training led to his repairing most of the cleft palate and harelip deformities in the Fort Smith area. [8]

His marriage in 1912 was recorded in the September 26 issue of the Fort Smith *Daily Herald*:

> Dr. Everett Foster, son of Dr. and Mrs. J.H. Foster, will be married October 9 to Miss Lynn Iler, a favorite society girl of Shreveport, La. Dr. Hunt will accompany Dr. Foster to Shreveport and act as best man at what will be one of the most fashionable society weddings ever held in the Louisiana city. After a trip to New Orleans, New York, Philadelphia, Atlantic City, and other eastern points the happy couple will return to Fort Smith and be "at home" at 501 North Eighteenth Street. [9]

(Liz Wolferman Haupert observes that this clipping confirms the impression of Mary Lynn Foster as a Southern lady, whereas her own mother, Elizabeth Moulton Wolferman, was more of a tomboy who hunted quail with her husband and taught him to fly fish—with dry, not wet flies. The two ladies were the best of friends.)

Among his other interests: the *Daily Herald* of Fort Smith reported in July 1913, that Dr. M.E. Foster's Tony Faust was second in the Class A Pace at the Matinee Club's fairgrounds meeting on July 4. [10] (Horse racing, including harness racing, had been popular in Fort Smith since the 1850s. Races were held at Spring Park, on

Racetrack Prairie, approximately where Ramsey Junior High School now stands. [11]) Dr. Foster later owned a ranch on the Fourche La Fave River and spent spare time there. He enjoyed fly fishing in Colorado with the Moulton and Wolferman families.

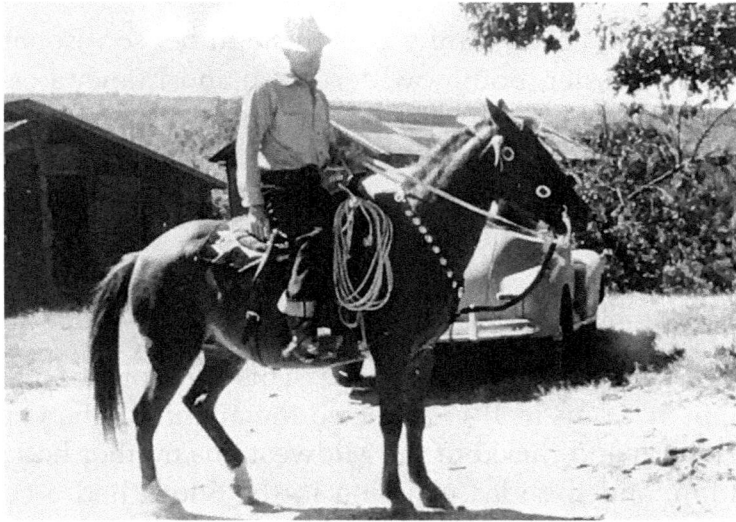

Dr. Foster enjoyed spending weekends at his ranch, the "Lazy F," often entertaining clinic and hospital staff there. (Photo courtesy of Cooper Clinic archives, Pebley Center, UAFS)

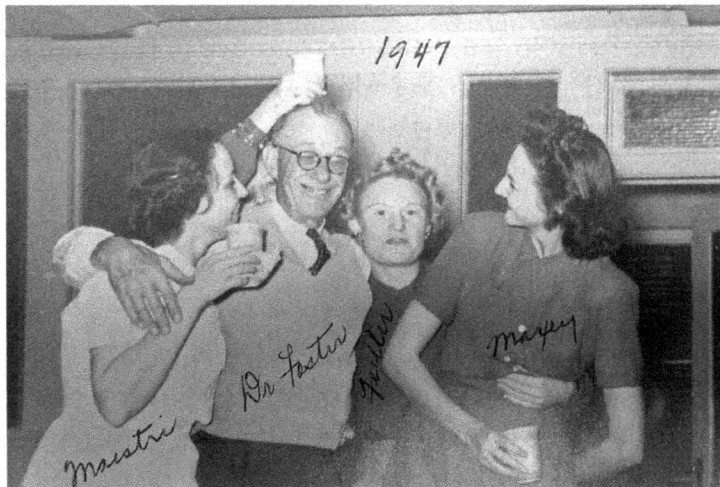

Everett Foster dropped his gruff operating room demeanor for a clinic party in 1947. A hidden face above his right shoulder must be responsible for the cup being held above his head. (Photo courtesy of Cooper Clinic archives, Pebley Center, UAFS)

Dr. Foster was forced to retire in 1963 because of peripheral vascular disease, which led to his death in 1966 at age seventy-nine. [12] He was survived by three children, Dr. Miles Foster, who was a pathologist in North Platte, North Dakota; Robert Foster of Fort Smith, who was retired from the United States Weather Service; and Eva Foster Whitehead of Houston, Texas. [13]

My connection with the Foster family was through his son Robert and Robert's wife Lenamae "Trip" Foster, both now deceased; and I fancy I can visualize Dr. Everett Foster with the characteristic facial features and voice that were passed on to both his sons. Much of the oral tradition about Dr. Foster was passed on to me by his office nurse, Ann Miller (whom he called by her maiden name "Polla"), when she was a nursing supervisor at St. Edward.

Sidney J. Wolferman

"Rural town in Arkansas needs physician." This note on the bulletin board at Barnes Hospital in St. Louis in 1913 attracted the attention of a young resident in training. Though born and raised in the Midwest, his mother had grown up on a Virginia plantation, and the idea of living in the South had a certain romantic appeal. He answered the notice, joined an older physician, and began his practice in Fort Smith. The young doctor was Sid Wolferman, whose uncle, Col. Joseph M. Heller, was an Army physician who had sent him stamps from a posting in the Philippines, giving him an early orientation toward a career in medicine. [14]

Sid Wolferman was born in Streator, Illinois, January 7, 1889, the son of David and Carolyn "Carrie" Frank (Heller) Wolferman. David had come with his family from Birchfield (Birkenfeld) in Rhineland-Palatinate, Germany. The family was Jewish but decided not to practice the Jewish religion or customs.

His mother Carolyn was Jewish and grew up on a plantation in Virginia. Carolyn's sister Ida Heller married Isadore Saks, who with his brother Andrew Saks founded the first Saks store, the predecessor of Saks Fifth Avenue.

Sid skipped a grade in Streator because he disrupted class. He received his BA degree at the University of Wisconsin, his MD at Northwestern University in Chicago in 1911; and he did his internship and residency training at Barnes and St. Louis City Hospitals in St. Louis. He was assistant to the dispensary physician of St. Louis and then moved to Fort Smith on October 1, 1913.

After a short time in practice with the older physician who had posted the notice on the hospital bulletin board, Wolferman elected to begin his own solo practice.

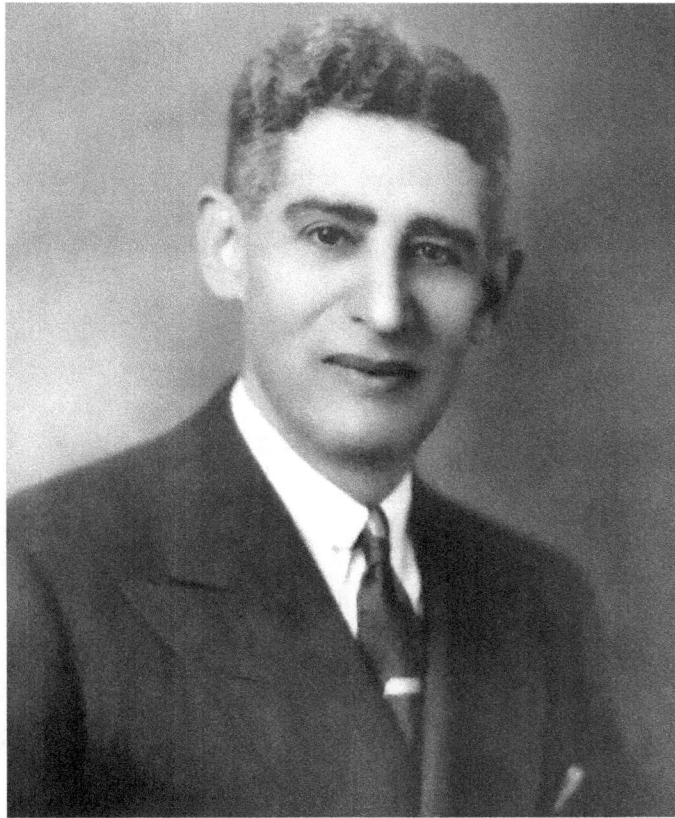

Portrait of Sidney Wolferman hangs in the old Cooper Clinic main lobby.

One can track some of his professional interests through short newspaper clippings. While still a resident at St. Louis City Hospital, the *New York World* quoted Dr. Sidney Wolferman, "insanity expert at the City Hospital," who reported that sixty-three cases of insanity had been admitted to the hospital in the month of January 1913, more than twice the monthly average. Dr. Wolferman ventured the opinion that one reason for this increase was the high cost of living, provoking a flurry of correspondence and editorial comment. [15]

As a Fort Smith physician, Dr. Wolferman quoted Dr. S.W. Harrison, "prominent negro physician of this city," as saying that "eighty-three percent of the negroes who live in Fort Smith are afflicted with tuberculosis . . . Dr. Wolferman urges the erection of a tuberculosis sanatorium for the negroes." [16]

The clouds of war were gathering, and a clipping of April 5, 1917, is headed, "Businessmen Practice Drill." [17]

Businessmen of Fort Smith gathered in force at the Plaza Wednesday at noon to enroll for the noon day civilian military drill. The conditions of the drill were explained to the crowd, namely that their services were voluntary and that in joining the squad no man assumed any obligation whatever.

Dr. S.J. Wolferman, who has been active in the movement since its inception, acted as enrolling clerk, and in a short time secured the following roster though many had no chance to sign who will sign when the squad meets at 6 o'clock Thursday afternoon to decide whether the drills shall occur three times a week, or daily.

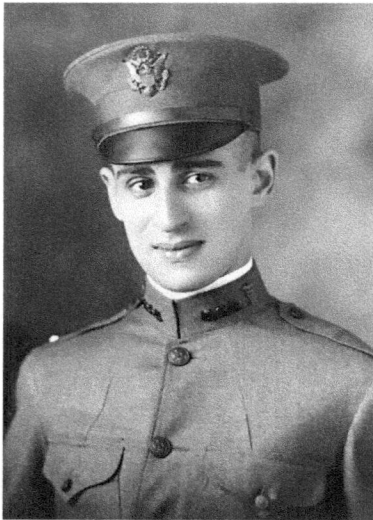

Sid Wolferman led Fort Smith businessmen in marching drills in early 1917, just prior to American entry into World War I. He volunteered for service and was commissioned a first lieutenant in the regular army medical corps, at age twenty-eight. (Photo courtesy of Liz Haupert)

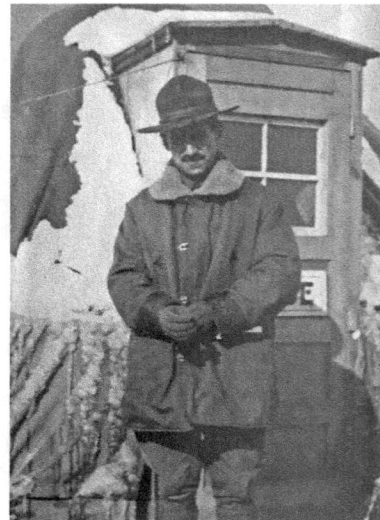

Lt. Wolferman had special training in plastic surgery during his service in World War I. (Photo courtesy of Liz Haupert)

When war came, Dr. Wolferman was commissioned as a first lieutenant in the regular army medical corps. Another clipping announces,

One of those wonderful opportunities which this world war is opening up on every side for young men of promise and ability has just come to the fortune of Dr. Sidney Wolferman, of Fort Smith, Arkansas. He has been appointed among thousands of young physicians who are to take a special course in Plastic and Oral Surgery, which is one of the most delicate and difficult of all phases of surgical work . . . Dr. Cooper of Fort Smith is responsible for Dr. Wolferman's name, which combined with the fact that Dr. Wolferman had worked under Dr. (V.P.) Blair, the world-renowned surgeon, gave him double recognition.

Dr. Wolferman will be sent to St. Louis at government expense, where he will study and conduct special experiments along this line . . . [18]

(As noted above, Dr. Foster also studied plastic surgery under the same Dr. V.P. Blair in St. Louis during World War I. After the war Dr. Foster seems to have made plastic surgery a personal specialty in Cooper Clinic. Dr. Wolferman became the clinic's primary orthopedic surgeon. He was also recognized as a diagnostician in internal medicine. Specialties did not appear to be so segregated at this transitional stage in medical history.)

During his military service Lieutenant Wolferman specialized in facial surgery at Fort Oglethorpe, Georgia; also serving at Camp Sevier, Georgia, and at Garden City, Long Island. He studied plastic surgery, orthopedic surgery, and radiology at the Army Medical School in Washington, D.C. [19] Early in his military career the young bachelor physician sent a letter home describing his experiences. Lacking wife or local family, he addressed his letter to the Fort Smith Rotary Club. These excerpts may be a bit graphic, but this is the way it was:

Camp Greenleaf,
Co. 8, Second Bat.
Fort Oglethorpe, Ga., Nov. 18,1917

Dear Jack and Fellow Rotarians:

I've neglected you all, but it is not due to the fact that I have not thought of you often, for I have, but camp life is not conducive to letter writing and we are kept well occupied.

When I first went to St. Louis, they worked us from morn until night and then we had to study in the evening. In that special work of "making new faces out of old," the war has developed much, and we had to go some to learn it. We were made first to do a dissection of the human head and neck, working out all nerves, blood vessels and muscles. All the little muscles of facial expression that in previous work we had paid no attention to, now had to be worked out in detail. After getting that down, the different operations, and their mechanisms were explained to us, and we were given cadavers and had to perform each operation. In order to make it even more practical (and though this is no secret it doesn't sound good for general talk) a number of cadaver heads were shot with .45s and we had to repair all injuries. The work is getting to such a degree that really, they could change Louis's nose to look like D.C.'s.

. . . I can't begin to tell you all the wonders of this place. But just draw upon your imagination—we are camped upon the famous Chickamauga Battlefield. Each morning we drill on the historic Kelly field, and twice a week have review on

McDonald Field. On a riding lesson last week, I rode all along Missionary Ridge and went up Lookout Mountain. That's the atmosphere we are in.

. . . The weather is fine about noon, but the mist settles in the evening and by night it's the coldest place on earth. It takes about 5 blankets and a comforter to keep warm--& it's sure cold when we turn out—Our only consolation is the little saying that everyone fires at you if you kick. "You're in the army now."

Hope you may be able to read this writing & that I have not bored you—My very best wishes to you all & to Rotary, I am—

Sincerely,
Sid [20]

Upon his return to Fort Smith, he became one of the original founders of Cooper Clinic. A century later, it's difficult to realize how revolutionary this concept was. The distribution of income among the partners was probably based on whatever system the Mayo Clinic used; and whether determined by the entire group, a compensation committee, or Dr. Cooper himself, it did not appear to be based solely on production. Liz Haupert recalls that in its beginning the clinic did one third of its work as charity. This was not a system for everyone, and it's worth noting that three of Dr. Cooper's original six partners left the group within five years, for one reason or another. During its first four or five decades, more physicians left the group than stayed with it. Time and money, in one form or another, prove to be recurrent issues, and a paragraph in the minutes of the Clinic meeting of March 23, 1924, is an example:

There was general discussion about loafing in the noon hours of doctors and getting back to work on time, and about Sunday afternoon work. It was agreed that everyone should eat lunch as soon as possible and when not busy to immediately come back to the Clinic. It was generally agreed that the men should sort of pair off, so that one out of each two would be available Sunday afternoons when necessary.

Everyone was advised to keep the front office informed as to where they were on their calls and when they left the building and when they arrived. [21]

It goes without saying that Saturday mornings were standard office hours.

The young bachelor physician became a somewhat older bachelor physician before finally marrying, in 1928 at the age of forty, Elizabeth Moulton, age twenty-eight, daughter of Dr. Everett Crockett (E.C.) Moulton, Sr., and granddaughter of Dr. Herbert Moulton, both ophthalmologists of Fort Smith. Dr. Herbert Moulton had set up his practice in Fort Smith in 1890. The new Mrs. Wolferman also had a brother, Everett, who was the third of four generations of Moulton ophthalmologists in Fort Smith. Sid joined his in-laws and the Fosters on annual vacations to Workman's Ranch in Greeley, Colorado, on the headwaters of the Rio Grande River. The children went along for two weeks in the summer, and Sid and Elizabeth went together for two weeks each fall.

The Colorado connection was significant in that Everett Moulton Jr. met his wife Bettye Tripplehorn when they were both fishing there; and Dr. Everett Foster's son Bobby met his wife "Trip" Tripplehorn, Bettye's cousin, at the same ranch.

Liz Haupert recalls that the doctors were a close-knit group socially as well as professionally. Dr. Cooper, though older, was a close friend and associate, and he and Dr. Wolferman bought a bank together in Oklahoma. That was in 1928, and it is not thought that the bank lasted very long after 1929. Bill Brooksher, radiologist at St. Edward, and his wife Peggy were close family friends. Dr. Foster, though not related, was "Uncle Everett."

Liz's older sister Linda was the last baby Dr. Cooper delivered: he died the next day, in 1930. Dr. Wolferman was called to the house, but Dr. Cooper died before he arrived.

Dr. Wolferman's favorite retreat was the ranch of Dr. Walter G. Eberle, with its biggest attraction: no telephone. Liz Haupert recalls that the telephone company provided her father with an extra-long cord so that he could keep a telephone on the dining room table; he answered every call himself, and the telephone company also provided him with a phone jack for a receiver in every room. This may not appear remarkable to those who always carry a cell phone with them, but Liz says she never saw so many telephones in anyone else's house.

Participation in organized medicine and in civic organizations were part of the responsibilities of a physician as Dr. Wolferman understood it, and he continued a variety of extracurricular activities—writing an article for the newspaper about the school system's responsibility to remember the physical health of the students and be alert for such deficits as poor vision; treating Jimmy Jamiski, star third baseman of the Fort Smith Twins, for the fracture of two small bones in the right ankle in 1920, as club physician; delivering a lecture to the Teachers' and Parents' Association of Belle Point School, on the care "necessary for an infant"; and serving on a technical advisory committee for the Arkansas Crippled Children's program. He was president of the Fort Smith Rotary Club in the later 1930s. [22]

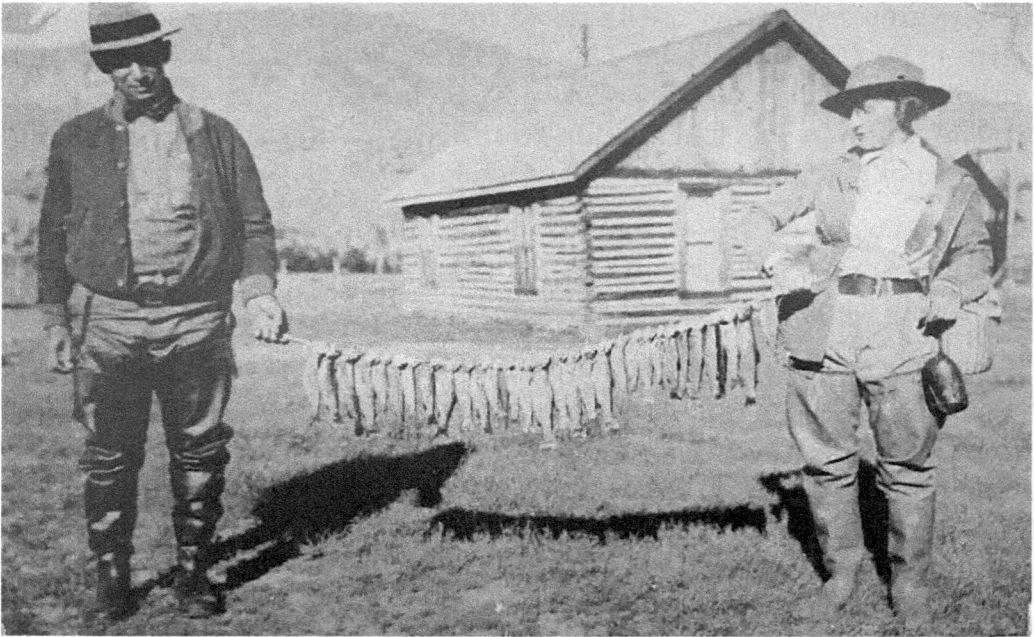

Elizabeth Wolferman, twelve years younger than her husband, taught him to fly fish in Colorado, where they spent vacations every year. Mrs. Wolferman died in Fort Smith at age 101. (Photo courtesy of Cooper Clinic archives, Pebley Center, UAFS)

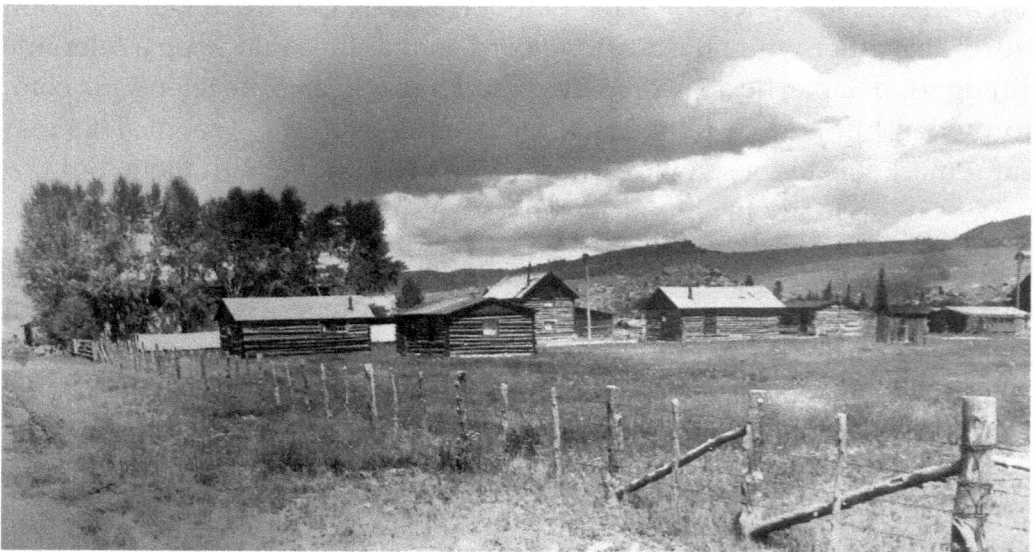

The Foster, Wolferman, and Moulton families vacationed regularly at this primitive ranch near Greeley, Colorado. Fly fishing was good, but there was no indoor plumbing. (Photo courtesy of Cooper Clinic archives, Pebley Center, UAFS

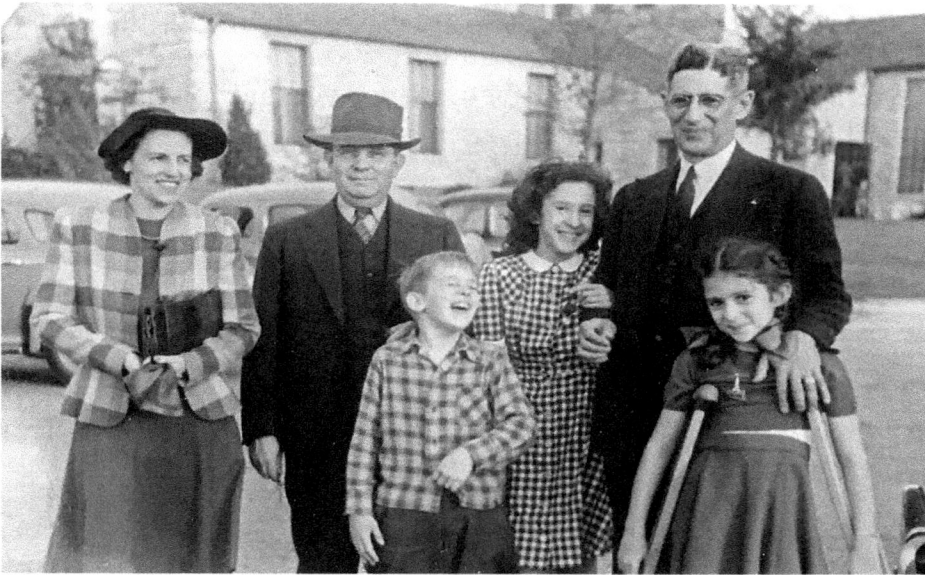

*The Brookshers and Wolfermans were close family friends. Peggy Brooksher, left, died in 1970. William Brooksher, in the hat, was Director of Radiology at St. Edward at the time of his death in 1971. He served as editor of the **Journal of the Arkansas Medical Society** from 1934 to 1954. Their only child, William R. (Bill Riley) Brooksher, III, was chief resident in internal medicine ay UAMS when he died in an automobile accident in Little Rock at age twenty-nine, after having been married for a week. Linda Wolferman was three years older than her sister Liz, on crutches, in front of her father Dr. Wolferman. (Photo courtesy of Liz Haupert)*

Professional honors and responsibilities included election as a Fellow of the American College of Physicians in 1928; directing the meeting of the Fort Smith Clinical Society in 1932 during his term as president, when he presented a paper on "The Evaluation of the Surgical Treatments for Peptic Ulcer"; serving as president of the Arkansas Medical Society in 1939; and serving as councilor of the Southern Medical Association.

Practice responsibilities were especially heavy for the doctors who were too old to serve in World War II. Dr. Wolferman had a heart attack in late 1944, spent six weeks at bed and chair rest, and stopped smoking, using Life Saver mints liberally. His daughter Liz recalls, "Only a few months before he died, he responded to a request for a house call by explaining that since his heart attack he was no longer able to make house calls. The woman said, 'Don't tell me your troubles, Dr. Wolferman. I didn't ask you to be a doctor.'"

"One night he called my mother to give him a shot in his stomach. I don't know what the shot was, but he died within an hour or two." He was fifty-six when he died on February 18, 1945. His funeral was at First Presbyterian Church.

Born of Jewish parents who did not identify with Judaism, he developed friendships both within the Jewish community and among non-Jews. He attended the Presbyterian Church with Elizabeth whenever one of the daughters was playing a part in the service, but otherwise "he was one of those who said he could find God on lakes and creeks," his daughter recalls. He loved the nuns at St. Edward, enjoyed taking them to Dr. Eberle's farm to ride horses, and every morning before making rounds at St. Edward he sat silently for a few moments in the chapel. Interestingly, he belonged to Hardscrabble Country Club decades before the club initiated a policy of welcoming Jews to its membership.

Irvin Sternberg quotes Mrs. Wolferman as saying that her husband "felt every pain that every one of his patients had." Liz recalls, "He was just a very happy person."

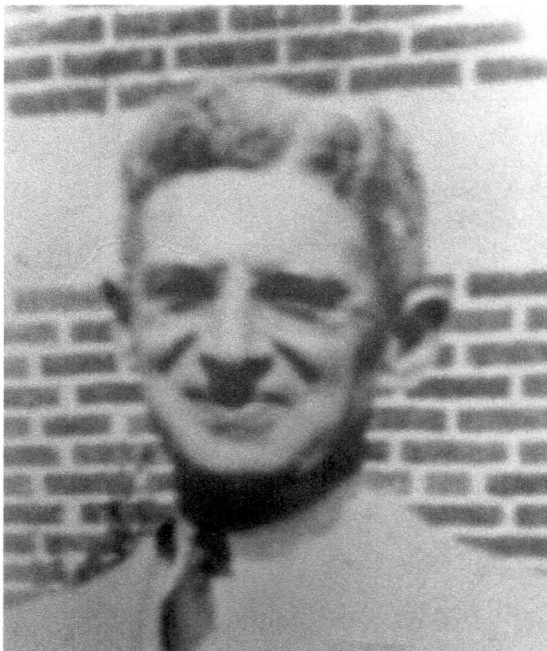

Dr. Wolferman is shown in an informal snapshot taken outside Cooper Clinic. "He was just a very happy person." (Photo courtesy of Liz Haupert)

Davis Woolf Goldstein

Dr. Davis Goldstein was the only founder of Cooper Clinic still living when I joined Cooper Clinic in 1969; he died in 1980 at the age of ninety-one. As a dermatologist, he was the only one of the founders to limit his practice to a defined area of specialization; but his sense of public service and private charity was wide. During the depression he personally underwrote projects to ensure that every child served by welfare had a Christmas present. [23]

Rabbi Sam Teitelbaum of the United Hebrew Congregation in Fort Smith walked through the lobby of Cooper Clinic in the late 1930s and was astonished to find black and white patients sitting together. He had never seen this before in the South. Dr. Goldstein, a member of the UHC, explained: "You, Rabbi, did this to me, and I did it to my colleagues . . . You motivated me to realize that 'colored people' are human beings and must be treated as such." [24]

Davis Goldstein was born to Marx and Rosa (Woolf) Goldstein in Greenville, Mississippi, September 14, 1888. After graduating from Greenville High School, he began studying pharmacy at Tulane University, but he changed his mind and enrolled at the University of Tennessee College of Medicine in Memphis, where he worked in a chemistry lab and in drug stores to pay tuition costs. He served as an intern at the John Gaston Hospital in Memphis, and since there were few options available for dermatology training in the United States, he spent eight months in 1910 touring dermatology centers in Europe, spending three months in Vienna and studying in London where he became acquainted with Sir Alexander Fleming, later the discoverer of penicillin. When in Paris he studied under Marie Curie, the discoverer of radioactivity. Upon his return to the United States, he worked at the Skin and Cancer Hospital in Philadelphia.

He came to Fort Smith in 1912 and practiced dermatology until World War I. He volunteered and served as Regimental Surgeon in the 328th Combat Infantry Division. (He knew Sergeant Alvin York, recipient of the Congressional Medal of Honor.) [25] Captain Goldstein was decorated for service under fire in the Meuse Argonne offensive, and in 1919 he was promoted to Major. [26]

After World War I, he and other veterans of the war—Drs. Foster, Wolferman, and Klingensmith—joined St. Cloud Cooper in forming the Cooper Clinic, where Dr. Goldstein's specialty was listed as dermatology and radium therapy. He was the only dermatologist in the clinic until Calvin Bradford, the first trainee to complete the dermatology training program at the University of Arkansas for Medical Sciences, joined him in 1963. Dr. Bradford, who referred to Dr. Goldstein as "one of the most honorable men I have had the privilege of knowing," was taken aback when he came to Cooper Clinic and Dr. Goldstein looked up at him and told him in his gravelly voice, "You and I are going to be married to each other."

Professional and community service were intertwined for Dr. Goldstein. He was chairman of the Sebastian County Department of Public Welfare for many years; helped organize the Arkansas and Sebastian County Cancer Society; coordinated the work of hospitals, nurses, and doctors of the Arkansas State Crippled

Children's Agency; and was American Legion post commander and served many years as chairman of the Legion's Child Welfare Committee.

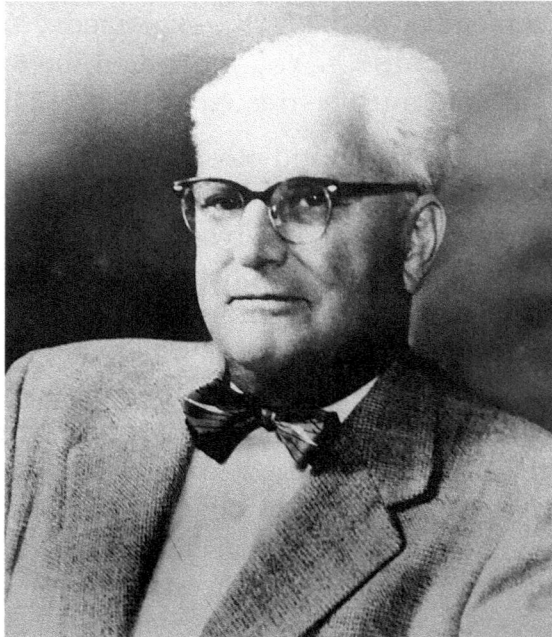

This portrait of Davis Goldstein hangs in the old Cooper Clinic main lobby.

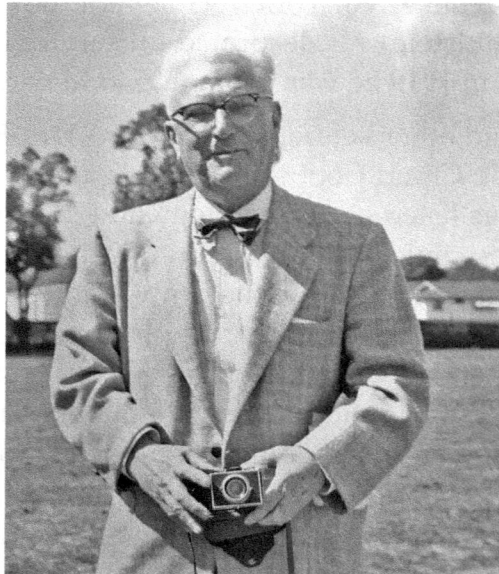

Shown here with a camera, Davis Goldstein continued to play an active part in the life of the community.
(Photo courtesy of Cooper Clinic archives, Pebley Center, UAFS)

The Davis W. Goldstein Dermatology and Research Fund was established by Dr. and Mrs. Goldstein in 1965. The gift to the medical center included his personal medical library of some two hundred volumes, funds to maintain and expand the new facility, and a continuing trust fund to further knowledge and research into diseases of the skin. [27]

As a diplomate of the American Board of Dermatology and Syphilology, he was the advisor to the local Health Department on the management of venereal disease at Camp Chaffee; and he worked in the health department's venereal disease clinic, at a time when syphilis was treated with weekly injections of bismuth and arsenic. [28] Less well known was his medical care for the women who worked at Miss Laura's and other houses of ill repute. His waiting room may have been racially integrated, but he had a separate entrance for these women so that they could come discreetly for diagnosis and treatment.

Active in the American Medical Association, he was vice president of the Arkansas Medical Society and president of the AMA's Fifty-year Club.

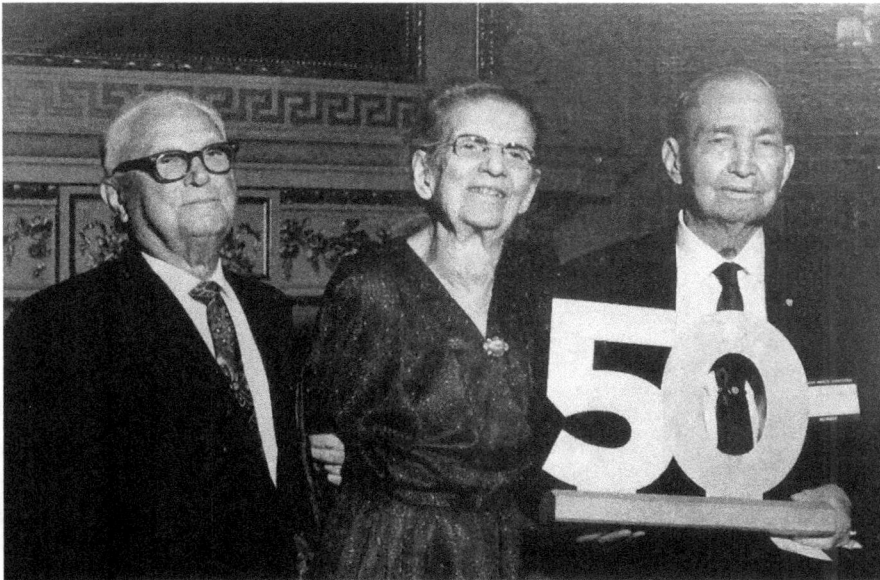

Dr. Goldstein served as president of the American Medical Association 50-year club. (Photo courtesy of Cooper Clinic archives, Pebley Center, UAFS)

The Fort Smith Noon Exchange Club honored him in 1954 with its Book of Golden Deeds Award. He served as president of the Fort Smith Rotary Club in 1934–1935, having been a member since his first arrival in Fort Smith.

He was active in the Jewish community and was president of the United Hebrew Congregation. Upon retirement from Cooper Clinic in 1969, he was given a set of golf clubs. He played regularly at the Fort Smith Country Club, which was a public golf course, and he continued to play well into his late eighties.

Davis Goldstein married Florence Pahotski, who came from a Fort Smith Orthodox Jewish family, in 1917. [29] They had one daughter, Gloria Goldstein Klein (1922–1984). Florence Goldstein died in 1973, and Dr. Goldstein subsequently married Leona (Farber) Heilbron, a longtime family friend who had lived in Fort Smith and had been away in California for some years. [30] She survived him by three years, dying in 1983.

(I remember Leona Goldstein with great fondness; she was a generous, loving person, and she gave great joy to Davis. On entering her hospital room at Sparks during an illness, I found them both laughing. "We've just been talking about old times and old friends," he explained.)

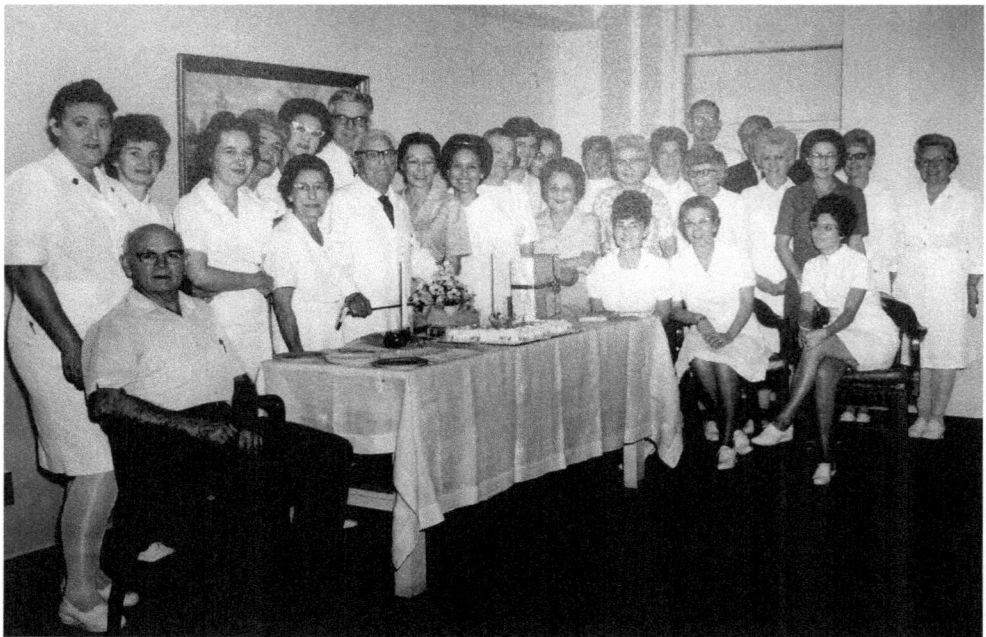

Dr. Goldstein is holding a golf club presented to him at his retirement in February 1969. Vi Wakefield, long time laboratory technician, stands left of Dr. Goldstein. Dr. Calvin Bradford, his partner in dermatology, stands behind him. Mary Ethel Ledbetter, longtime clinic office manager, in an off-white dress, stands right of Dr. Goldstein. Cooky Sadler, surgery office nurse, stands beside Mrs. Ledbetter. Dr. J.V. LeBlanc, clinic internist (in glasses) and J.L. McAleb, clinic manager, stand in the rear to the right. (Photo courtesy of Cooper Clinic archives, Pebley Center, UAFS)

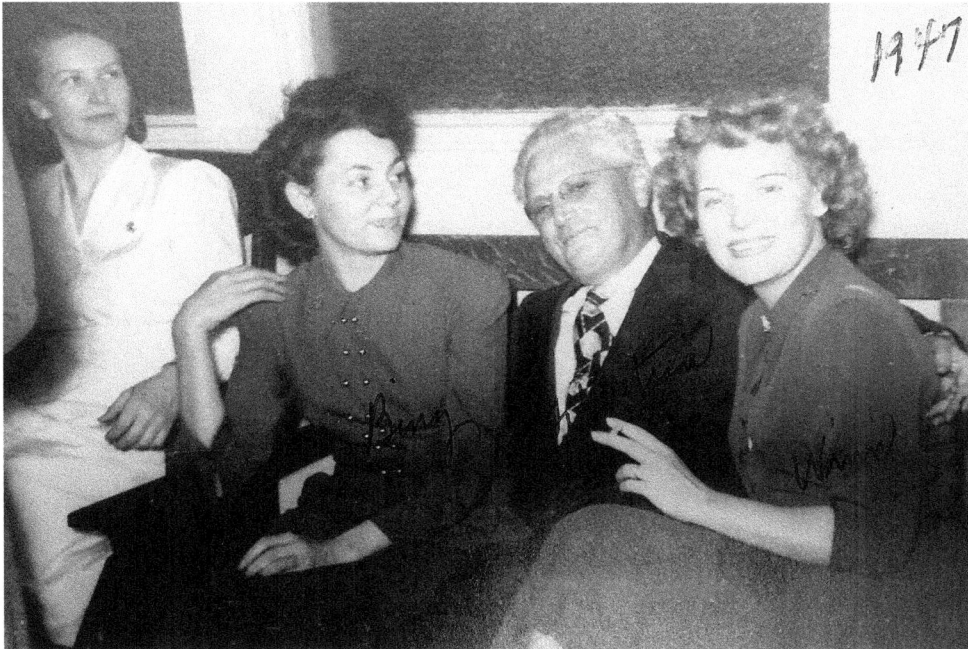

The Goldsteins enjoyed entertaining clinic staff in their home for New Year's parties. (Photo courtesy of Cooper Clinic archives, Pebley Center, UAFS)

Arless A. Blair

Dr. A.A. Blair was born in Scranton, Arkansas, in 1891; attended Paris High School, the University of Tennessee, and the University of Tennessee College of Medicine; did an internship at St. Mary's Hospital in Hoboken and a residency at St. Louis City Hospital; served as captain in the Medical Corps in World War I; and came to Fort Smith to practice after the war. [**31**]

Dr. Blair's name first appears in the minutes of Cooper Clinic in an entry of March 14, 1921, when it was agreed that work "previously referred to Sparks Memorial Hospital" be referred to Dr. A.A. Blair "incident to the absence of Miss Owens from the Hospital." A subsequent entry of November 28, 1921, shows that Dr. Blair would be named director of the clinic laboratory. It was decided to make Dr. Blair an offer to come into the clinic at the meeting of January 23, 1923. "It was decided he do inside work and be trained as assistant to Dr. Thompson. Percentage he was to be offered will be decided later. Dr. Foster was to tell Dr. Blair." The matter of his joining the clinic was discussed at several subsequent meetings through June 18, 1923, with "no definite action taken."

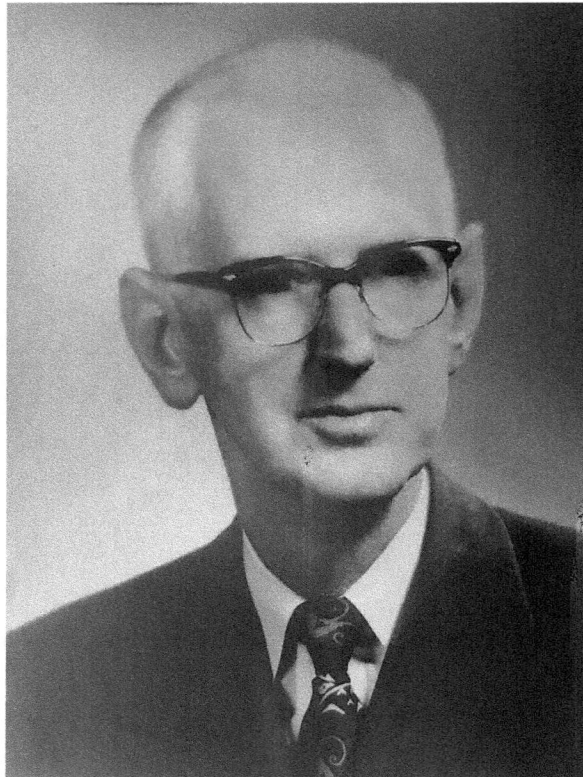

A. A. Blair, shown in this clinic portrait, became a partner in the clinic three years after its founding and shifted the emphasis of his practice from laboratory medicine to internal medicine. He served as governor for Arkansas of the American College of Physicians, and he served on the Fort Smith school board for eleven years.

Minutes are unaccountably lacking for the second six months of 1923, but apparently Dr. Blair was officially taken in as a partner during this time. An undated "analysis of sale" shows assets to be transferred in connection with Dr. Blair becoming a member. A schedule of payments by Dr. Blair to the clinic shows the first of five annual payments to be made January 1, 1924. [32]

It appears that Dr. Blair emphasized pathology and laboratory supervision in his early years but then changed his practice to internal medicine after joining Cooper Clinic. He went on to practice in the clinic until his untimely death October 24, 1955, at age sixty-four. He served as president of the Sebastian County Medical Association and was governor for Arkansas of the American College of Physicians. He served on the Fort Smith school board from 1935 to 1946 and was president of the Sebastian County TB Association. He married Florence Ware McKennon of Fort Smith in 1919, and they had two daughters. [33]

Cooper Clinic

The definitive step that identified Cooper Clinic as a proper clinic was the move to a new building at the corner of Little Rock Avenue (now Rogers Avenue) and 13th Street in 1924. The clinic consisted of two floors, as described by Dr. Ken Thompson in a 1990 clinic anniversary celebration: "The basement of the clinic (in 1939) had parking space for five cars for the founders—two Lincolns belonging to Drs. Foster and Wolferman, a Cadillac for Dr. Blair, and Dr. Goldstein's Dodge, which was parked nearest the door, since he didn't drive well in reverse. Dr. (William) Adams and I parked outside." [34]

For whatever reason (following the custom of the day, they were smokers), most of the founding pillars died relatively young, most of them still working—Dr. Cooper in 1930 at age sixty-nine; Dr. Wolferman at age fifty-six in 1945, Dr. Foster at age seventy-nine, in 1966, after a three-year retirement because of peripheral vascular disease. Dr. Goldstein (though shown in one photograph with a cigar, he must not have smoked very many of them) enjoyed a vigorous old age and retirement. Among other things, he took classes at Westark Community College. With his death in 1980 at age ninety-one, an era passed.

While these doctors were pushing forward in private medical care in Fort Smith, another era in management of one of the area's, and the world's, major diseases came and went. These changes, centered in Booneville and Fort Smith, will be described next.

A Breath of Fresh Air

Sanatorium Care for Tuberculosis in Arkansas

Having grown up with the comfortable assumption that there's an antibiotic for everything that handwashing doesn't prevent, it's hard for us to imagine the fearful place that tuberculosis held in the thought world of our forebears just over a century ago—especially those whose families included someone in an upstairs bedroom afflicted with the disease. This chronic infection caused one in seven deaths in Arkansas in the early twentieth century; some eighty per cent of those with active disease succumbed. [1] "Consumption" primarily involved the lungs and caused the victim to wither away slowly, sometimes suddenly coughing up large quantities of bright red blood. It was mostly managed in the home, somewhere out of sight of casual visitors.

Treatment of this widespread agent of death made its way from the home to the institution in the twentieth century with the establishment of sanatoria, often in remote isolated areas—such as the Arkansas Tuberculosis Sanatorium in the wooded hills a few miles south of Booneville. The concept of management in an isolated place with fresh air, healthy nutrition, and an opportunity for prescribed rest and exercise had moved from Europe to the United States in the late 19th century and to Arkansas in 1909 with passage of Act 378 by the General Assembly, creating a board of trustees to locate a suitable site. [2] The first patient was admitted to the new Arkansas Tuberculosis Sanatorium in October 1910, and by the end of the year there were sixty-four patients in residence. The Booneville facility was for white patients, though the incidence of tuberculosis was higher in the black population. With no sanatorium care available to black patients, two African American doctors in Little Rock provided small frame houses for their tuberculosis patients. [3] The Thomas C. McRae Sanatorium, a twenty-five-bed facility for black patients, was opened in 1930, in Alexander, Arkansas. The two separate sanatoria were combined in the Booneville unit in 1967 because of federal integration policies, and the McRae site was then used for other purposes. [4]

Special accommodations were made for children on the Booneville campus. A children's building was constructed by the Belle Point Masonic Lodge of Fort Smith in 1924, and a school on the campus was built in 1927. An expansion program in 1930 brought the total patient capacity up to 200, but the waiting list grew to as many as 300 with a four- to six-month wait before admission. [5]

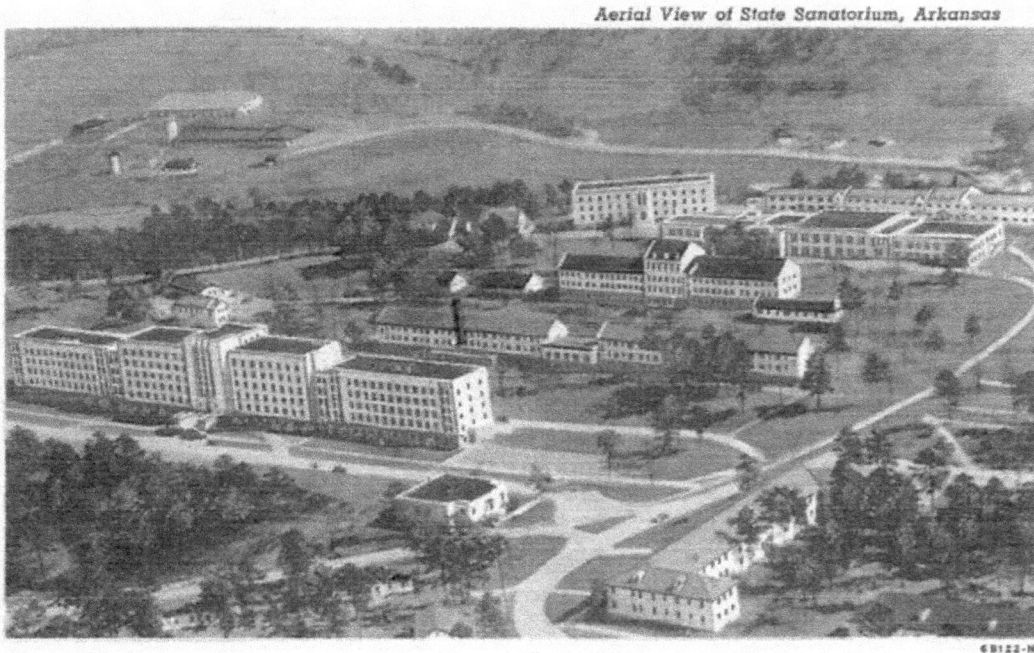

This postcard shows the extent of the sanatorium campus near Booneville. (Photo from Koon, D: "Every day was a Tuesday," **Arkansas Times***, June 2010)*

The Wildcat Mountain Annex

The need for beds in Booneville in the 1930s was so urgent that the Board of Control of the State Tuberculosis Sanatorium looked beyond the Booneville campus to an eighty-acre site east of Fort Smith that had been used by the WPA (Works Progress Administration) to house transient workers during the Depression. By that time the Wildcat Mountain camp included "nine or ten buildings with stone foundations and a brick veneer nurses' home and physicians' home" on a thirty-acre segment of the eighty-acre site. [6]

The WPA provided funds to construct four more buildings, allowing the facility to accommodate one hundred patients. A postcard image from this period shows thirteen buildings, including two three-story structures on the east side of the property (the back side, furthest from Wildcat Mountain Road).

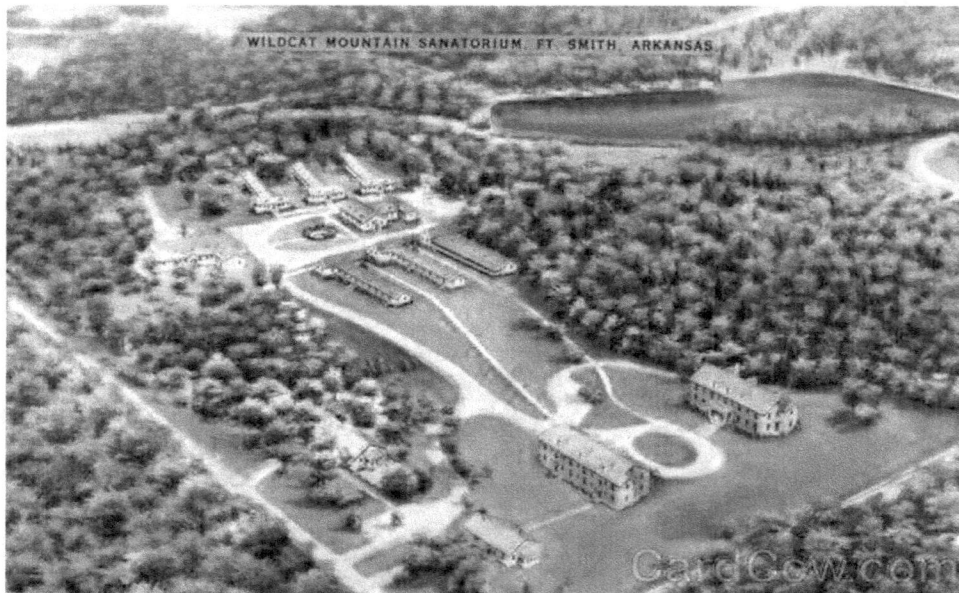

A 1930s postcard shows an aerial view of Wildcat Mountain Sanatorium. Wildcat Mountain Lake, now the Carol Ann Cross Lake, is at upper right. Wildcat Mountain Road, now 74th Street, is at the top, and Euper Lane is on the left. (The author found this postcard in a used book shop in Seattle, Washington.)

The first forty-three patients arrived on March 26, 1937, and the Wildcat Mountain Annex was soon filled. [7] It was used primarily for advanced and terminal cases.

Joseph Chalmers Irwin II (1888–1958) was a patient at Wildcat Mountain Sanatorium, though not as a terminal case. Working as an engineer in the Panama Canal Zone, his sore throat was diagnosed as tuberculosis of the throat. He returned home to Fort Smith in 1946, was admitted to Wildcat Mountain Annex, and then transferred to Booneville. With streptomycin newly available for treatment of tuberculosis, he transferred in 1949 to a private sanatorium in Shreveport, Louisiana, for treatment. He then returned home in 1950 as an arrested case. He discovered, however, that his friends would not see him because of fear of catching tuberculosis. Returning to work at the state highway department did not work out well because his friends and colleagues there were afraid to be around him. He finally decided to return to the Wildcat Mountain Sanatorium as an arrested case where he counseled patients. His wife said he was doing a lot of good there, and this provided him a social outlet. A room at the sanatorium was his home during the week, and then he returned home to be with his wife on weekends. He died in 1958 at the age of seventy. [8]

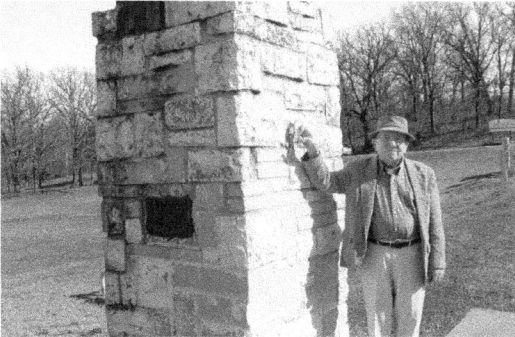

Joe Irwin, whose father had tuberculosis and was a resident at the Wildcat Mountain Sanatorium, holds one of the two rings that held the chain across the entrance to the grounds. This pillar and the one across from it on Euper Lane formed the entrance to the camp and are all that is left of the original WPA construction. (Photo by author)

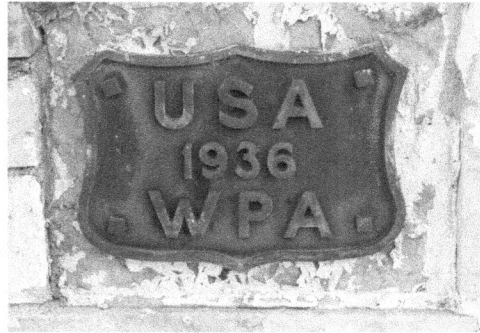

This plaque on one of the two pillars marking the entrance to the Wildcat Mountain grounds indicates that the WPA established these two pillars at the entrance to the camp in 1936, the year before the camp for transients closed and the Wildcat Mountain Sanatorium was established. (Photo by author)

The Nation's Largest Sanatorium

The hundred beds at the Wildcat Mountain annex, however, made only a drop in the bucket in view of the great need for sanatorium beds, and the Arkansas General Assembly provided the funds for a major addition in Booneville in the 1930s—but only under the prodding of a young legislator from Helena, Arkansas, who was himself a victim of tuberculosis. Leo Nyberg, barely in his thirties, got out of his sickbed in 1938 to lead the fight for a two and a half-million-dollar building program to the Arkansas Tuberculosis Sanatorium. [9] Sadly, Nyberg died at the Wildcat Mountain Annex in 1940, at the age of thirty-four, before completion of the building named in his honor. This was the Nyberg Building: 521 feet (a tenth of a mile) long and five stories high, housing 511 patients. In time the Booneville campus would house as many as 1,110 patients at one time and would become known as the nation's largest tuberculosis sanatorium. [10] In addition to over a thousand patients, some three hundred staff members lived on the site.

The sanatorium in Booneville became a self-sustaining city, with a campus that included dormitories, staff entertainment buildings, a chapel, a laundry, and a water treatment plant, with its own farms and fire station, orchards, school and newspaper.

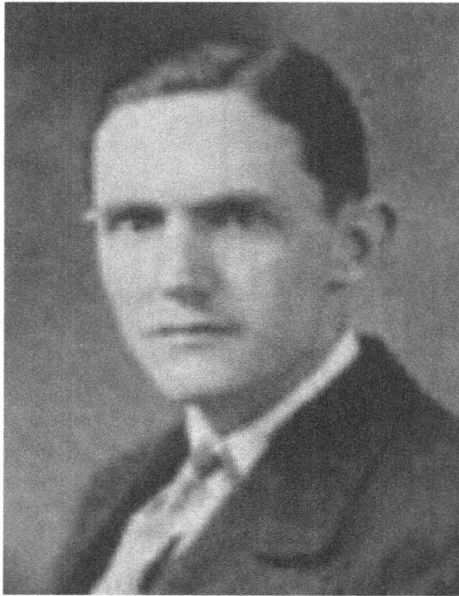

Leo Nyberg, state congressman from Helena, promoted measures for dealing with tuberculosis in Arkansas and died of tuberculosis at Wildcat Mountain Sanatorium in 1940, at the age of 34. (Photo from Findagrave web site)

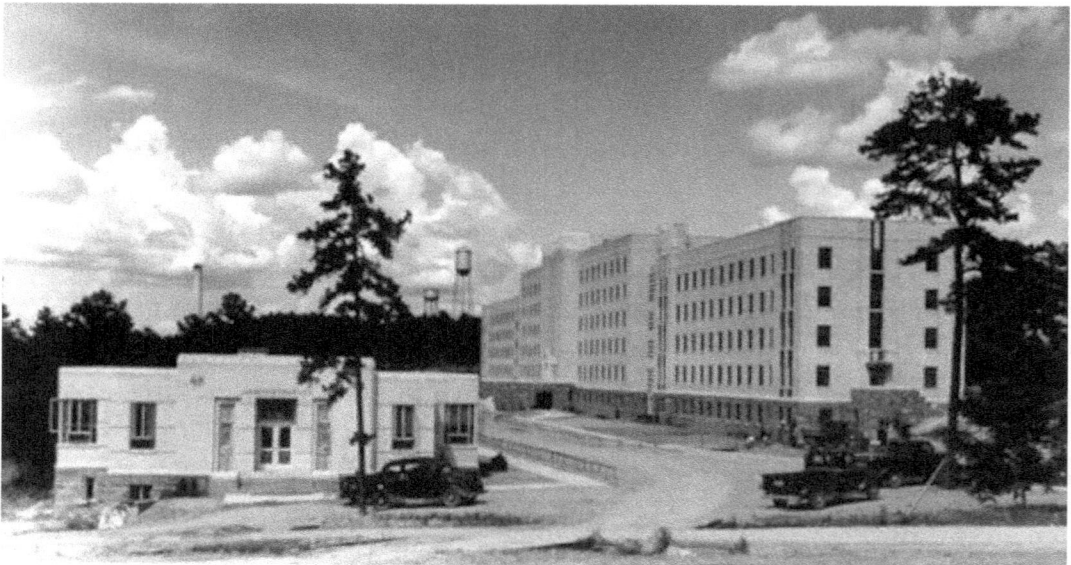

*With completion of construction of the Nyberg Building, the Arkansas State Tuberculosis Sanatorium became the largest in the nation. (Photo from Koon, D: "Every day was a Tuesday," **Arkansas Times**, June 2010)*

With the patients confined to the grounds and much of the staff living on the campus, the sanatorium was a world of its own, a way of life that has become the subject of imaginative fiction such as *The Hill* by Kevin Johnson (Tipsy Mockingbird Books, LLC, 2018). In this time-travel story, a present-day visitor to the deserted floors of the Nyberg Building finds himself going back in time to the heyday of the sanatorium, becoming a participant in the life of the community. *The Magic Mountain*, written in 1924 by Thomas Mann, who won the Nobel Prize in 1929, is the classic fictional account of sanatorium life. As he begins his stay at a facility high in the Alps, Hans Castorp is told by one of the other residents, "They make pretty free with a human being's idea of time, up here. You wouldn't believe it. Three weeks are just like a day to them. You'll learn all about it . . . One's ideas get changed."

The experience of being a sanatorium patient in Arkansas was like that of the fictional Hans in the Swiss Alps. Richard Myers was seventy-three years old when he told a reporter about being picked up by a big black car that carried him from his family's sharecropper shack on a farm in eastern Arkansas to the hills on the other side of the state. Although he had no symptoms, he had a diagnosis of tuberculosis involving his left lung. He would not see his family again for four years. [11]

Living alone in a room on the third floor of the Nyberg building, Richard began to lose his concept of time. "Every day in our lives was a Tuesday," Myers said, "because nothing ever happens on a Tuesday." Fresh from a farmhouse with no electricity or running water to an institution that provided those amenities and all the good food he could eat, Richard was transferred to the children's building—the "Masonic Building"—where he attended school with the other children four hours a day. But it was scary.

> "I suppose the worst part was the dying. That was a part of your existence. People died almost daily. I can remember laying there in bed at night, listening to people down the hall. It always began with a long coughing spell, then it would turn into a kind of gurgling, raspy sound. Then it would get deathly quiet. You knew what had happened."

After seven years of treatment, Richard was discharged at age fourteen and later served twenty-two years in the Air Force. "I was totally institutionalized by the time I was fourteen years old." He moved back to Booneville after retiring from the Air Force and went to work on the grounds of the old sanatorium, by then closed and functioning as the Booneville Human Development Center. But he had mixed feelings about the site. "To me, I think the place should be torn down and forgotten," he said. "It was a terrible place. I don't know why you would want to remember that much suffering and death and devastation—why you would make a monument out of that. It destroyed thousands and thousands of lives."

Every story was different. Donna Abraham was a nursing student at Kansas City General Hospital in 1945 (the same year that Richard Myers was admitted to the Booneville sanatorium) when she became acutely ill with fever, night sweats, and chills. [12] A diagnosis of tuberculosis was made, and it was later learned that she was one of ten students on a cancer unit who had contracted tuberculosis while caring for a patient who was later found at autopsy to have had tuberculosis, not cancer. The student nurses' duties had included suction of the lungs. Though she could have entered a sanatorium in Kansas, her parents preferred Booneville because it would be only 120 miles from their home in Siloam Springs. She was transported to the train station in Kansas City by ambulance with siren wailing, but she was able to sit with other passengers in the coach car because she was not coughing and therefore considered not infectious.

Once in the sanatorium, the chief enemy was boredom. Rest, wearing a sleep mask for two hours every morning and two hours every afternoon, was required. Meals were brought to the room, and lights were turned out at 9 p.m. Her roommate, more seriously ill, was not allowed out of bed. Donna was seriously bored. However, in a matter of a few months she improved enough that she was moved to a building for ambulatory patients. Here she slept on a veranda at night, and she was allowed to go about the campus for meals, movies, and visits to the store.

Donna was discharged after two and a half years and went on to become a public health nurse.

And Then It All Changed

The Arkansas sanatorium became a national leader in introducing new methods of treatment such as thoracoplasty, in which some ribs are removed to shrink the lung volume and collapse any cavities, and pneumothorax, in which air is injected into the pleural space to collapse the lung. These radical procedures would soon become obsolete, however, with the appearance of such drugs as streptomycin, isoniazid (INH), and para-amino salicylic acid (PAS) for the treatment of tuberculosis, starting in the 1940s. These agents were so effective that patients could be treated in general hospitals and at home. Having spent two months of my internship in a tuberculosis sanatorium in North Carolina in 1963, I was surprised to find in the 1970s that tuberculosis patients were treated on the regular medicine floor at St. Edward, in rooms identified by an ultra-violet light for protection against spread of air-borne germs.

I had missed a revolution that had begun in Arkansas in the 1960s. Drs. Joe Bates, Paul Reagan and William Stead had followed the evidence that led them to use the new anti-tuberculosis medications to treat patients in local hospitals, briefly, and at home for the rest of the time. Bates studied an outbreak of tuberculosis in the Arkansas Negro Boys Industrial School. By visiting the school and diagramming the spread of the outbreak in the dormitory, he concluded that the spread of tuberculosis was from tiny droplets, not from larger bits of sputum—confirming findings in laboratory animals that tuberculosis was not spread by close contact. An ultra-violet light could attack these droplets and make a room safe. [13]

Meanwhile, there was a gap in treatment of tuberculosis as patients were beginning to leave the sanatorium against medical advice. Sanatorium policy was to not prescribe outpatient medications for those who left against advice. Into this gap stepped Dr. Paul Reagan, Director of Tuberculosis Control for Arkansas, and Hermione Swindell, nurse consultant in tuberculosis to the Department of Health, setting up chest clinics throughout the state so that tuberculosis patients outside the sanatorium could be followed and treated. [15]

Based on the favorable results with treating outpatients in India, the Jefferson Memorial Hospital in Pine Bluff began treating tuberculosis patients in the hospital, initiating treatment in the hospital and discharging the patient after two weeks. At this point the patients were no longer infectious. [16] These results opened the door to hospital treatment of tuberculosis and marked the end of the era of sanatorium care. Ironically, the state that had been among the leaders in moving tuberculosis care from the home to the sanatorium was also one of the states to lead the movement from the sanatorium back to the home.

The Arkansas Tuberculosis Sanatorium remained open until 1973 when seven patients, the last of the 70,000 who had been residents in the Booneville sanatorium since it opened in 1910, were discharged. On June 30, 1973, the main gate was left unlocked for the first time in sixty years. [17] The facility is now the Booneville Human Development Center, occupying part of the first floor of the Nyberg Building. The upper four floors are vacant.

And the Wildcat Mountain Annex? Like other tuberculosis sanatoria, its census declined in the 1950s, and in 1952 space was made available for "elderly, destitute citizens" to be moved from the Sebastian County Hospital—otherwise known as "the county poor farm"—located on the present site of the University of Arkansas at Fort Smith, to Wildcat Mountain. [18] The thirty residents from the County Hospital were housed in a separate building on Wildcat Mountain, but the occupancy declined rather quickly, and this use of the sanatorium did not last very long. The Wildcat Mountain Annex for the treatment of tuberculosis closed its doors on December 1, 1958. [19]

Yet another use for Wildcat Mountain was found when the North Arkansas Conference of the Methodist Church built the Methodist Nursing Home on the site in 1961. [20] Independent living was added to the campus in 1974; and in April 2019, an outburst of community support led to the addition of an assisted living unit with a special section for memory care.

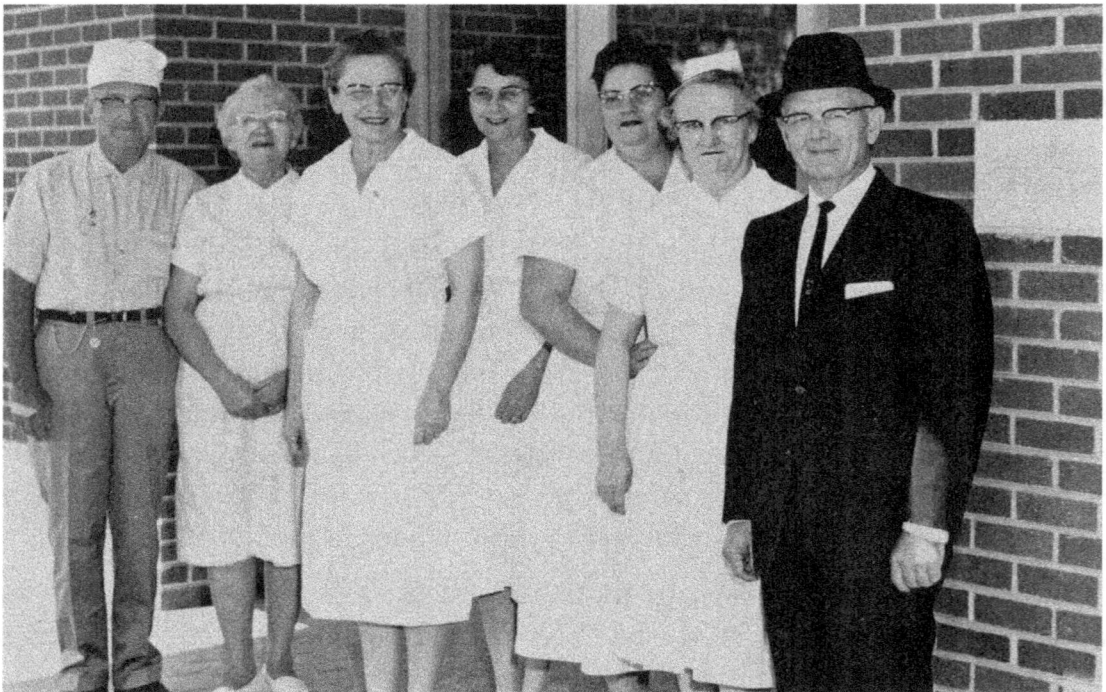

Hugh Wolfe, at right, was administrator of the Methodist Nursing Home when it opened in 1961. His wife, standing beside him, was the registered nurse. Other staff members are standing at the entrance of the facility. (Photo from Methodist Nursing Home opening ceremony brochure, 1960)

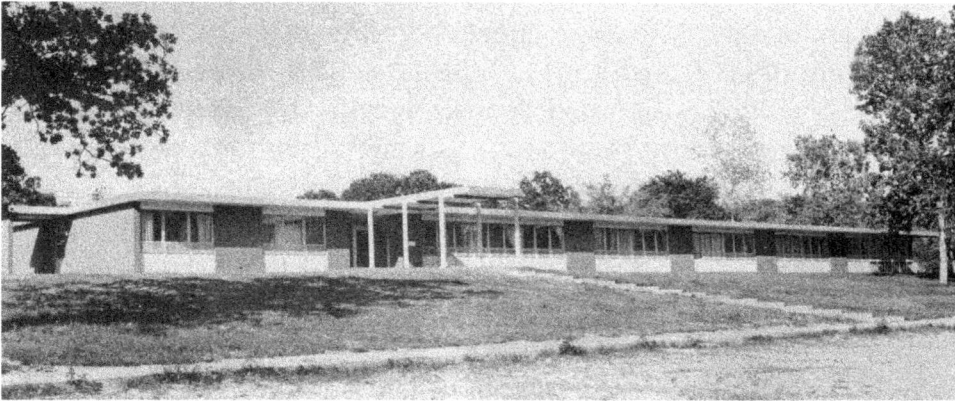

The Methodist Nursing Home received its first resident on March 19, 1961, with 33 beds: 15 double rooms and 3 single rooms. (Photo from Methodist Nursing Home opening ceremony brochure, 1960)

Looking Back at the Sanatorium Era

Times changed, and tuberculosis management moved on. Did sanatorium care work? Opinions are divided. One would intuitively assume that the chances for survival for someone with unhealthy living conditions would be improved by removal to a sanatorium that provided the healthiest surroundings that human ingenuity could improvise. Supporting this view, the article about the Arkansas Tuberculosis Sanatorium in the online *Encyclopedia of Arkansas* states that sanatorium care reduced the death rate from eighty per cent to ten percent. [21] However, one retrospective review states, "In the final analysis, the death rate in sanatoria or at home were the same—about half of patients died whether they were treated in a sanatorium or not treated at home." [22] Reliable figures are hard to come by. A controlled study of sanatorium care versus home care would probably have been considered unethical. In any event, there is no universally accepted evidence to settle the issue.

Considering sanatorium care in the context of the great number of cases of tuberculosis, one must not forget that sanatorium care only reached a small fraction of those who were afflicted with active tuberculosis, significantly diluting the impact of the institutions. And it is of interest that the number of cases and of deaths from tuberculosis began to decline in the early twentieth century, well before the revolutionary introduction of antibiotics in the 1940s; this decrease has been attributed to improvements in sanitation and living conditions. [23]

Yet the sanatorium movement did provide some unanticipated benefits. The subspecialty of pulmonology—diseases of the lungs—was born in tuberculosis sanatoria. When I began attending chest conferences in the 1960s, specialists in tuberculosis were often referred to as "phthisiologists"—an arcane term coming from Hippocrates, who designated "consumption" as "phthisis." In time these phthisiologists morphed into pulmonologists and spilled out of the sanatoria into academic health centers and private practice, specializing in all diseases of the lung, including emphysema, asthma, and cancer of the lung.

A recent visit to the Booneville Human Development Center showed the campus to be intact, almost looking like a college campus at spring break. The pillars of the gate are still there, but the arch between them bearing the name, "Arkansas Tuberculosis Sanatorium," is no longer to be seen.

And yet tuberculosis continues to be a world-wide killer, second only to Human Immunodeficiency Virus (HIV) as an infectious cause of death; almost a third of the world's population harbor a latent or active form of the disease. Organisms resistant to multiple drugs make it more difficult, and more expensive, to eradicate the disease.

Largely for these reasons, tuberculosis is far from being eliminated in the United States. The number of cases is decreasing, but 9,105 persons with tuberculosis were reported in 2017, the lowest on record. [24]

The fight will be carried on in this country without sanatorium care. The last remaining sanatorium in the United States, the Holley Sanatorium in Florida, closed in 2012. [25]

The tide had turned in the care of tuberculosis during the middle of the twentieth century. But this was also the time of a big, big change: World War II. The end of this war led to the return of doctors who had served their country in wartime, leading to a flowering of medical care that will be described next.

Postwar Renaissance

It was the era of penicillin. It was the era of World War II. It was the era of medical specialization. It was the middle of the twentieth century. And it was during this time that well-trained, highly competent young physicians came to Fort Smith from different parts of the country. Mixed with some remarkable home-grown talent, this aggregation of physicians came back from the war and established Fort Smith as a referral center that made the new advances in medical practice and technology readily available in the area.

Several forces came together after the war to create a medical renaissance in Fort Smith. The basic ingredient was personnel, and a survey of the profiles of the newcomers shows that many came to Holt-Krock Clinic, some to Cooper Clinic, where numbers would increase in later years, and quite a few occupied independent practices. A comprehensive survey of all these physicians is beyond the scope of this book; indeed, Amelia Martin has already done that in *Physicians and Medicine: Crawford and Sebastian Counties, Arkansas 1817-1976*, which contains biographical sketches of them all. A few stories, however, illustrate the changes that transformed the delivery of health care in Fort Smith.

In retrospect, a major reason for the influx of talent that made Fort Smith such a formidable regional referral center appears to have been the recruitment efforts of Dr. Fred Krock. Young doctors were certainly not traveling to Fort Smith from the nation's training centers because everyone knew about it. Somebody recruited them. For example, John "Swede" Olson (1912-2007) was recruited by Dr. Krock, who wanted a Mayo Clinic-trained surgeon. Dr. Olson met this requirement: after graduating from the University of North Dakota, he received his MD from the University of Pennsylvania in 1938 and interned at Presbyterian Hospital in Philadelphia. He trained in surgery at Mayo Clinic and received a BS degree (surgery) there in 1944, before serving as a ship's doctor in the U.S. Navy from 1944 to 1946. Dr. Krock found him in Philadelphia.

His daughter Sanna told me that after her father visited Fort Smith, he called her mother Clemmie (whose grandfather, a pharmacist, had patented Hires Root Beer) in Philadelphia and told her that Fort Smith was a nice place. Her mother, having grown up on Philadelphia's Main Line, had questions about anything west of the Alleghenies and south of the Mason-Dixon line.

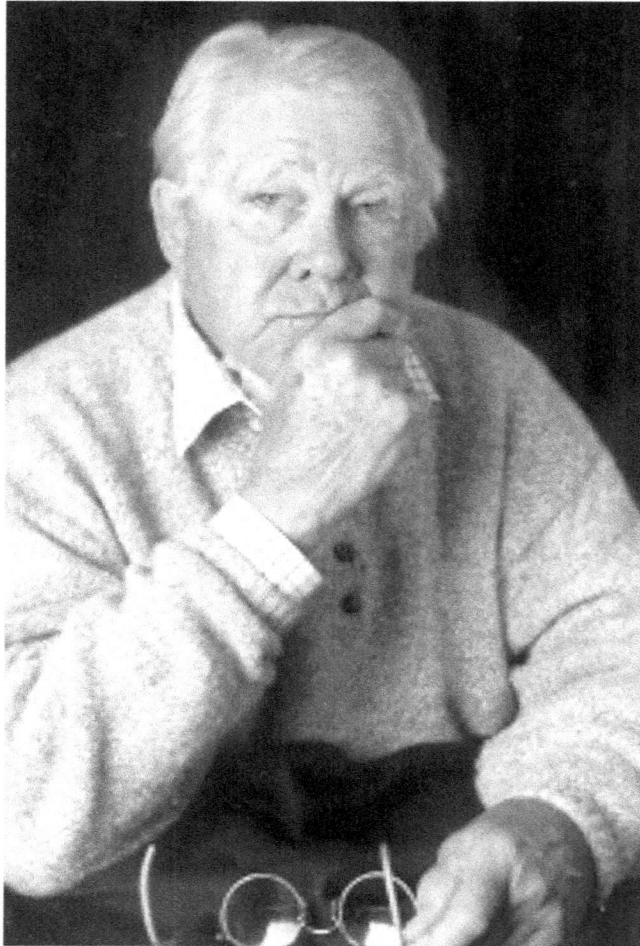

John (Swede) Olson (1912-2007) (Photo from Find a Grave website)

"Where is it?"

"It's in Arkansas."

"Where is Arkansas?"

"It's in the South."

"The South. Do they have palm trees?"

Dr. Olson practiced at Holt-Krock from 1947 to 1994, retiring at age eighty-two and living to be ninety-five. During this time the Holt-Krock surgery department developed a full complement of subspecialties.

Carl Wilson had already come in 1940 and established the urology department. Born in Yonkers, New York, in 1911, Dr. Wilson was a member of Alpha Omega Alpha, the scholastic honor society for medicine, at the University of Virginia, and he came to Fort Smith from Springfield, Massachusetts. After seeing action in Okinawa as a lieutenant colonel in the U.S. Army during World War II, he returned to Holt-Krock, where his brother Mort joined him in 1953, and his son Steve joined him in 1974. He was a member of the United Hebrew Congregation in Fort Smith, participated in a variety of community activities, and was active in clinic management.

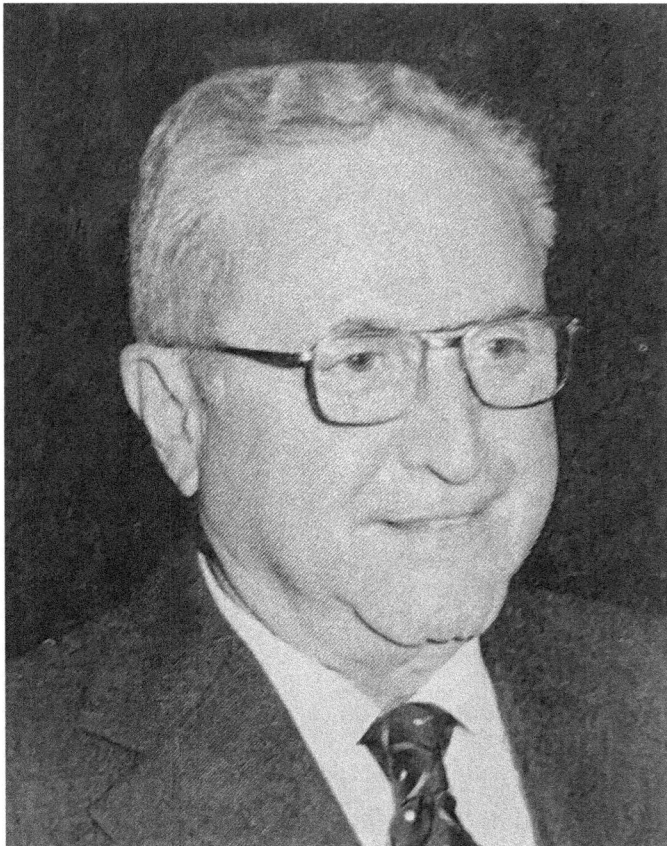

Carl Wilson (Photo from Physicians and Medicine: Crawford and Sebastian Counties 1817-1976, by Amelia Martin, 1976)

Another young physician who came south after serving in World War II was Albert S. "Bud" Koenig (1915-2007), who established his pathology practice in Fort Smith in 1946 after discharge from the army as a Captain. He grew up in Newark, New Jersey, graduated from Columbia College in New York in 1936, and received his MD from Columbia College of Physicians and Surgeons in 1939. After training in surgery at St. Luke's Hospital in New York City, he worked in industrial medicine for the E.J. DuPont Company in Old Hickory, Tennessee before serving in the U.S. Army from 1942 to 1946, working in the Clinical Laboratory at Camp Shelby for three years and then in the Twelfth Army Medical Laboratory of Saipan in the Mariana Islands.

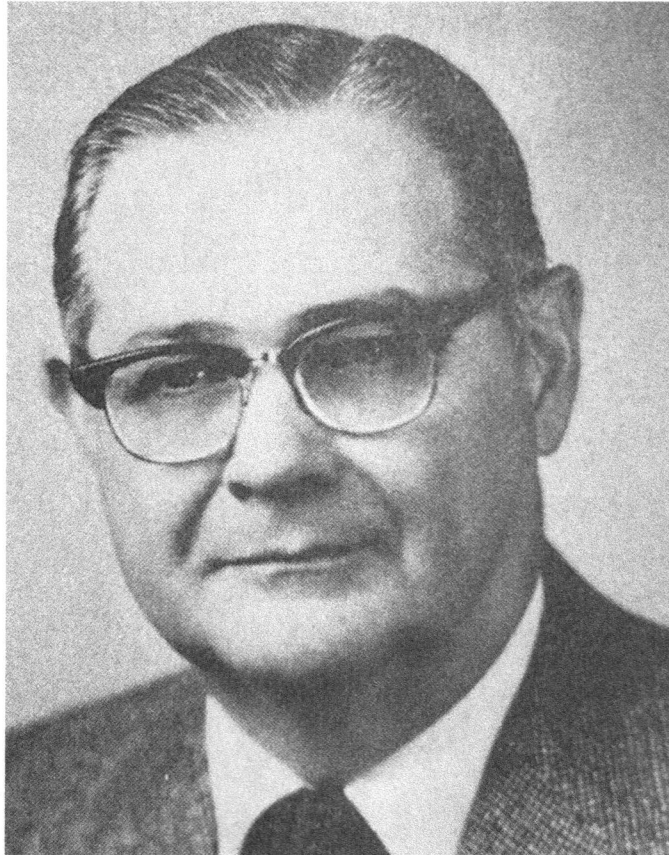

A. S. "Bud" Koenig (1915-2007 (Photo from Physicians and Medicine: Crawford and Sebastian Counties 1817-1976, by Amelia Martin, 1976)

He became the pathologist and director of laboratories at Sparks, St. Edward, and Crawford County Hospital in Van Buren, and he organized his own pathology group that later included his son Sam Koenig. Active in professional and civic leadership, he served as a governor of the College of American Pathologists, president of the Sebastian County Medical Society, councilor of the Tenth District of the Arkansas Medical Society, and trustee of Arkansas Blue Cross and Blue

Shield. I remember his broad smile as he celebrated his German heritage by leading the Rotary Club in singing "O Tannenbaum" at Christmas time.

As a young physician in Fort Smith, I was fortunate whenever I looked for x-rays in Sparks Radiology and happened to see Ernie Mendelsohn, who was invariably kind and appeared happy to visit with me. Dr. Mendelsohn had begun the radiology department at Holt-Krock and Sparks Hospital in 1941. He was born as the son of a pediatrician in Berlin in 1912, received his MD from the University of Berlin, and managed to stay in Germany as a Jew until finishing his internship at Jewish Hospital in Berlin. He was then able to get out of Germany and make his way to the United States where he completed a residency in radiology at Mount Sinai in 1941 before coming to Fort Smith.

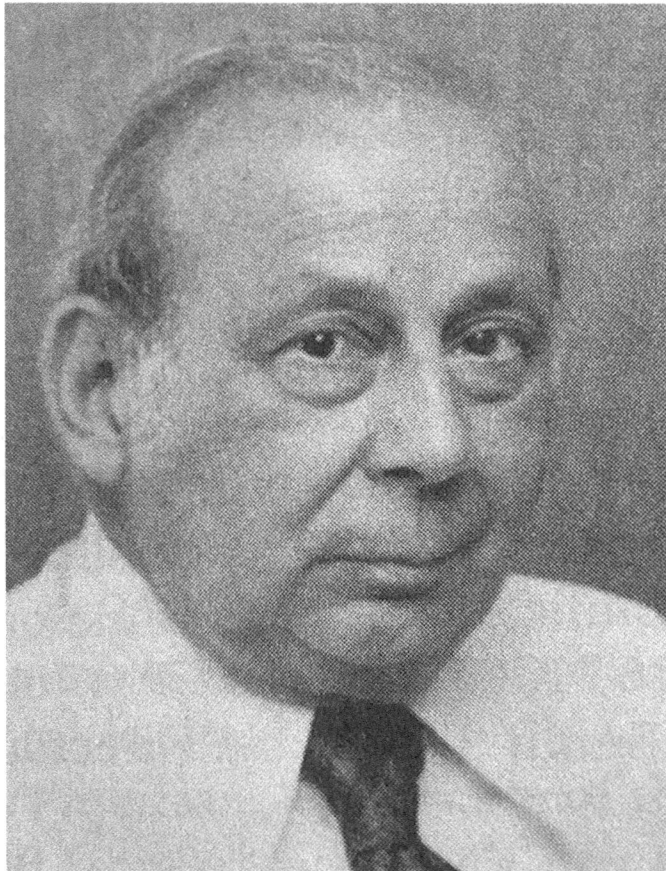

Ernest Mendelsohn (1912-1979) (Photo from Physicians and Medicine: Crawford and Sebastian Counties 1817-1976, by Amelia Martin, 1976)

105

Dr. Mendelsohn served as president of the Arkansas Radiological Society and of the Sebastian County Medical Society. He was associate clinical professor of radiology at the University of Arkansas for Medical Sciences and published several scientific papers during his time of practice. Civic activities included board membership in the Fort Smith Symphony Association and Fort Smith Art Center. He also served as president of B'nai B'rith in Fort Smith.

A photograph of W. R. Brooksher (1894-1971), with a ten-gallon hat, broad grin, and large cigar, hung in the St. Edward radiology department, which he founded, for many years. A native of Fort Smith, he joined his father, W. R. Brooksher Sr., a specialist in surgery and x-ray therapy, in practice in 1920. He was active in the Arkansas Medical Society, serving as its secretary for nineteen years and as editor of the *Journal of the Arkansas Medical Society* from 1933 to 1954. During this time the Arkansas Medical Society office was in Fort Smith. In his honor, the Arkansas Medical Society established a scholarship fund in the names of him and his wife Peggy for medical technology students in 1958. Their only child, Dr. William R. Brooksher III, died tragically in an automobile accident in Little Rock in 1962, a week after getting married.

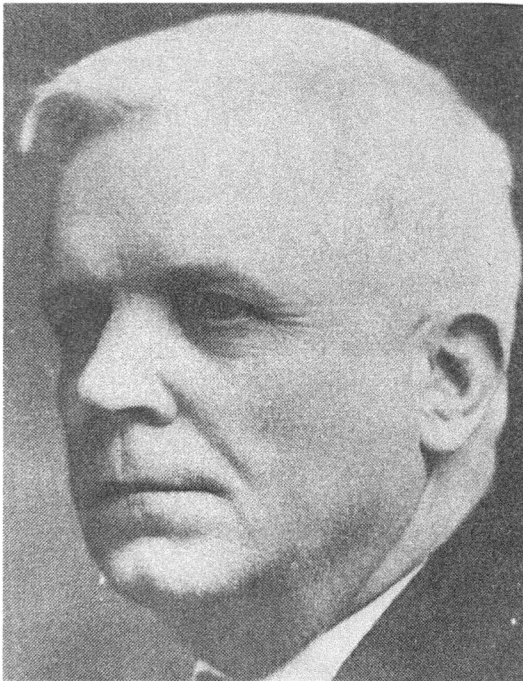

W.R. Brooksher, Sr. (1894-1971) practiced in Fort Smith from 1895 until his death in 1926. He was president of the Sebastian County Medical Society in 1900 and served on the school board. (Photo from Physicians and Medicine: Crawford and Sebastian Counties 1817-1976, by Amelia Martin, 1976)

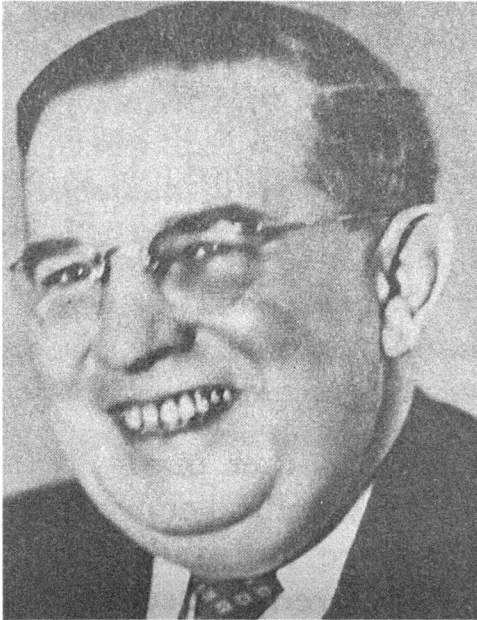

W. R. Brooksher, Jr. entered practice with his father in 1920 and practiced radiology until his death in 1971. (Photo from Physicians and Medicine: Crawford and Sebastian Counties 1817-1976, by Amelia Martin, 1976)

Another native of Fort Smith was Everett C. Moulton Jr., who was the third of four generations of Moultons to practice ophthalmology in Fort Smith. His grandfather Herbert Moulton (1861-1951) came to Fort Smith in 1890, where he practiced until 1940, serving as president of the Arkansas Medical Society in 1925 and contributing to several medical journals. Everett Jr.'s father, Everett Crockett Moulton (1889-1952), joined his father in practice in the early 1920s. The third of this line was Everett Jr., who joined his father in 1948. Like his father, Everett Jr. was an honor student at Northwestern University Medical School and a member of Alpha Omega Alpha. He trained at Massachusetts Eye and Ear, the Harvard teaching hospital in Boston. He was the one I knew, and although he was the soul of kindness, some of my greatest moments of anxiety were when I saw him for his annual physical examination and was obliged to use my ophthalmoscope to peer into Dr. Moulton's eyes. Like his father and grandfather, he continued to see patients in his office into his later years.

The Moulton Clinic was very much a family affair. When I came to Fort Smith in the late 1960s, Everett Jr.'s mother Juliette Gates Moulton, in her eighties, came to the office every morning and clipped names from the day's obituaries and then removed the name from the clinic files. Several ophthalmologists joined Dr. Moulton in his practice.

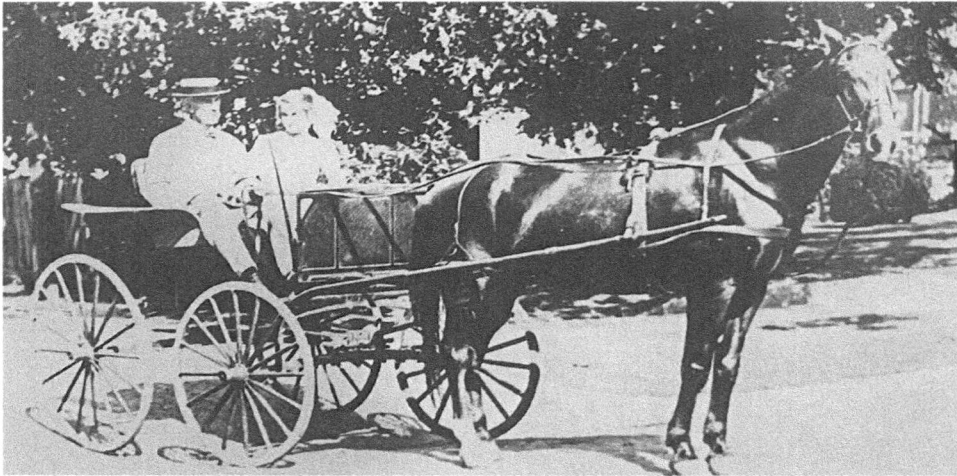

Herbert Moulton 1861-1951, grandfather of Everett C. Moulton, Jr. 1916-2008, with his daughter Elizabeth Martha (Photo from Fort Smith: An Illustrated History, by O.B. Faulk and B.M. Jones, Western Heritage Books, 1963)

Like his father who had served in World War I, Everett Jr. served in World War II as a medical officer, joining his troops as a Captain in the Fourth Cavalry in the invasion of Europe, receiving a Bronze Star.

His son Dr. Everett (Kit) Moulton then became the fourth of the line to practice ophthalmology in Fort Smith when he joined his father. His daughter Dr. Allyson Moulton. in turn, has returned to Fort Smith where she practices general surgery.

Of the two senior partners in Cooper Clinic when I arrived, Wright Hawkins was the one who played the role of keeper of the torch, the one who attended to the standards of the clinic and upheld them as an example for the newcomers. Dr. Hawkins was successor to Dr. Foster as the senior surgeon in the clinic. Dr. Foster, in turn, had been the one who filled in on at least one of the cases scheduled by Dr. Cooper himself on the day after the founder's death.

Dr. Hawkins grew up in Fort Smith, and his father Sumpter Hawkins was the pharmacist at one time in Cooper Clinic. Wright's grandfather Ichabod Wright Hawkins was a farmer and businessman who owned extensive cotton farmland in the Fort Smith area in the early 1900s and went to his "office" every morning in the Main Hotel next door to the First National Bank. Several local businessmen started the day with a shave in the hotel barbershop and then moved to the hotel lobby where there were three rows of large, overstuffed leather chairs. Each man had his own chair, not to be occupied by anyone else, and here the business of the city was conducted. [1]

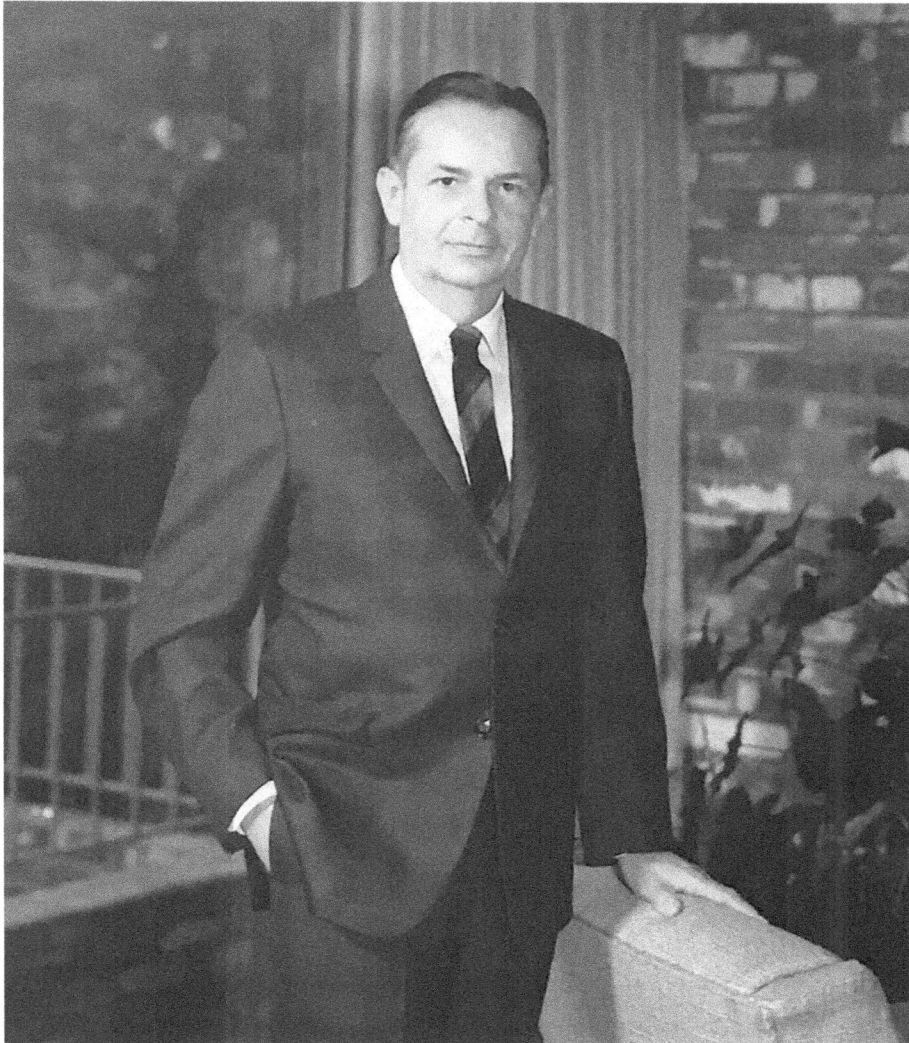

Wright Hawkins (1913-1983) (Portrait from Cooper Clinic)

Wright Hawkins attended Fort Smith High School, Fort Smith Junior College, the University of Arkansas, and Tulane University School of Medicine. During the war he was assistant chief of surgery at the 315th Station Hospital in Axminister, England; after his military service he did a surgery fellowship at Lahey Clinic in Boston before joining Cooper Clinic. He served as president of the Sebastian County Medical Society, published papers in the *Journal of the Arkansas Medical Society* and the Louisiana state medical journal, and he was on the Fort Smith school board for eight years.

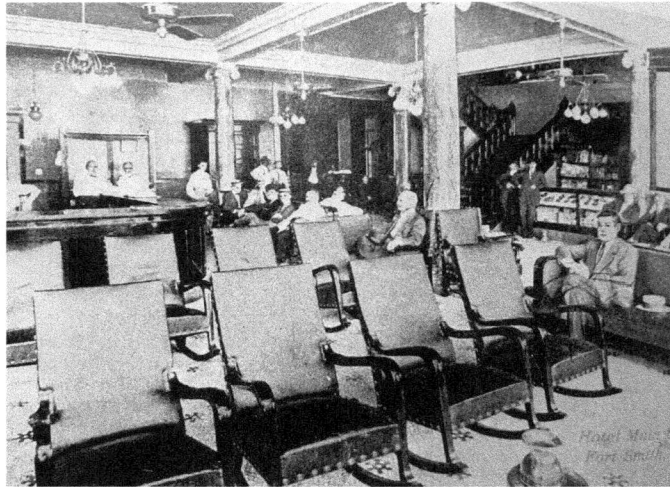

I.F. Wright, grandfather of Dr. Wright Hawkins, was one of several local businessmen who routinely conducted their business with one another in the lobby of the Main Hotel, next door to First National Bank which still stands on Garrison Avenue. (Photo from Fort Smith: An Illustrated History, by O.B. Faulk and B.M. Jones, Western Heritage Books, 1963}

His patients took his word as law. One word was sometimes enough, as with one of his patients who told me he had stopped smoking. How did he do it? "Dr. Hawkins told me to." I found this interesting. Dr. Hawkins had not yet quit smoking himself.

"What did he say to you?"

"I asked him if I should stop smoking. And he said: 'Yes.'"

Wright saw to it that we kept up appearances. We wore tuxedos when we hosted the clinic's annual Christmas party. He made sure that I joined the Rotary Club and that my wife Mary joined a particular women's organization that his wife Jayne belonged to. Jayne was a faithful partner who provided flowers for the new clinic building on Waldron Road for years, and who prepared full scale dinners for strategically selected guests. Wright was a genial host on these occasions, but he maintained his customary discipline. Promptly at ten o'clock he put down his after-dinner liqueur, cleared his throat, and stood up. "It's ten o'clock; I know we all have to go to work tomorrow."

Ken Thompson, the other senior partner in Cooper Clinic in the 1960s, was more of a free spirit. Though a dapper dresser, he was known for sometimes not wearing socks—even though the sight of a young doctor in the hospital wearing white socks would draw a quiet and private but rather snide comment from him.

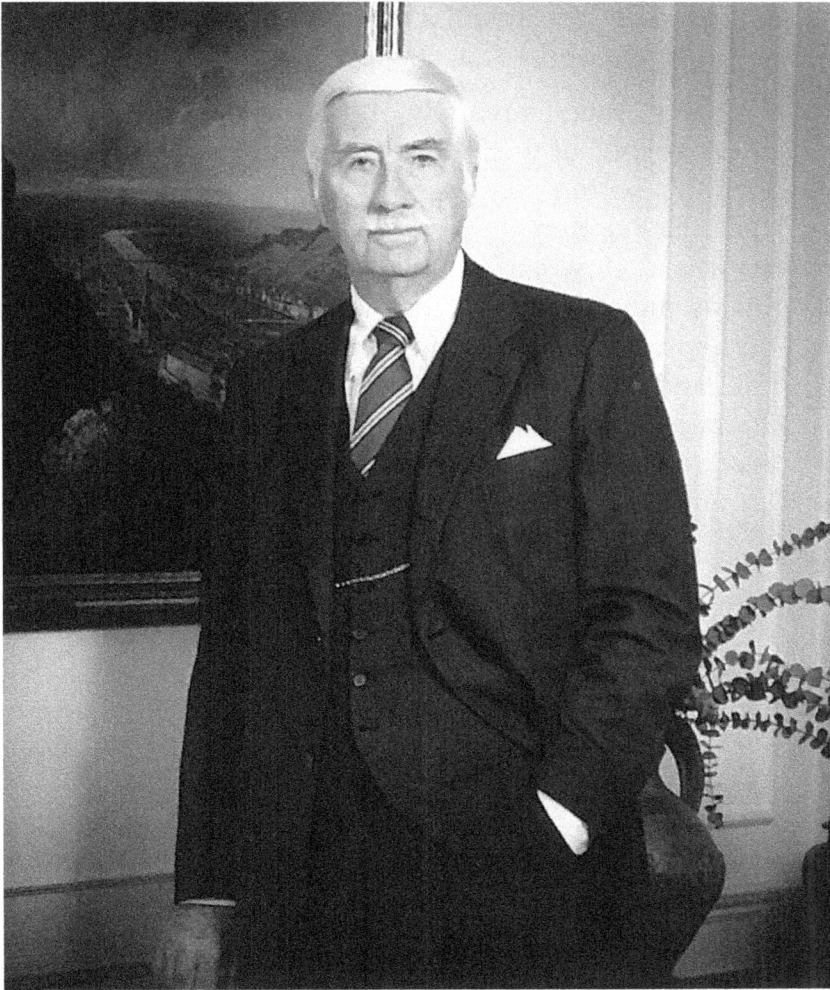

Kenneth Thompson (1911-1988) (Portrait from Cooper Clinic)

Dr. Thompson was born in 1911 and grew up in Princeton, Missouri; he was a sprinter on his high school track team and attended Westminster College on a track scholarship. As a singer in a dance band, he transferred to Louisiana State University on a music scholarship. Scholarships were given to his entire dance band so they could play with the University symphony. He then entered the University of Missouri medical school, at that time a two-year pre-clinical medical school, in 1934. A year later he was awarded an anatomy fellowship and served as assistant professor of anatomy, doing research on the connections of the thalamus in rhesus monkeys. He received an MA in anatomy in 1937 and transferred to Northwestern University School of Medicine. His MD was not awarded until he completed an internship at City Hospital in St. Louis in 1940. He then did one year of residency in neuropsychiatry at State Hospital Number 2 in St. Joseph, Missouri.

One of Ken's classmates at the University of Missouri was Miles Foster, Jr., son of Dr. Miles Everett Foster, one of the founders of Cooper Clinic. Ken met his future wife, Virginia Henton, whom Ken described as a beauty queen in Missouri, through Miles's wife Helen. Ken and Virginia were married in Fort Smith in 1937. Their honeymoon was a "slow trip to Chicago in a 1934 Ford with a rumble seat" for Ken to begin his junior year at Northwestern. Ken and Miles planned on practicing together, but World War II interrupted this plan. Miles was called to active duty in 1942 and spent five years at Fort Leonard Wood as a pathologist. The doctors at Cooper Clinic did not think they needed a full-time pathologist, so Miles Foster moved to Omaha, Nebraska, where he remained at Bishop Clarkson Hospital until retirement.

Meanwhile, Ken Thompson joined Cooper Clinic in July 1941, with a starting salary of $300 per month. He had planned to go into neuropsychiatry in St. Joseph, but he said that he became discouraged by the wards full of patients with neurosyphilis whose disease was incurable. He wrote a short memoir ten years after his retirement in which he described how he entered the army: "The clinic founders were veterans of World War I, and with all the Camp Chaffee activity in 1941, the partners felt that the clinic should be represented in the army. Since I was the newest and youngest, I seemed the logical one to represent us. I volunteered in January when my second daughter was six weeks old." He was sent to Europe as commander of a medical company in the 11th Armored Division, "which got me there just in time to participate in three campaigns (Ardennes, Rhineland, Central European), free the prisoners from the death camp at Mauthausen (May 6, 1945) and meet the Russians in Linz, Austria." He received a Bronze Star and returned to Cooper Clinic in December 1945.

He restricted his practice to internal medicine when circumstances permitted; but in his early years he delivered babies when obliged to do so, and on weekends he assisted Drs. Foster and Wolferman in surgery. He worked crossword puzzles quickly; and he approached diagnostic problems with the same enthusiasm for problem solving. Making diagnoses without benefit of CT scans and batteries of blood tests was a challenging exercise, and he loved sharing and discussing diagnostic possibilities. He was one of those who always gave the patient all the time they wanted, and I would know he was through for the day when I'd hear him bellowing down the hall, "Drop your shovels!"

He was my consultant of choice, particularly with neurologic problems, which he considered to be his subspecialty. He retired in 1977 and spent his last months in a senior living center in San Bernardino, California, near his daughter Dana. I last saw him there when we were visiting nearby for a family wedding. He died September 4, 1998. There was a reception in the fellowship hall of St. John's Episcopal Church after the funeral service, and as I was leaving, his youngest daughter Kay rattled a glass with her knife and said she wanted to read a clipping. It was about a high school track meet in 1929, when Ken Thompson, son of Mr. and Mrs. J.M. Thompson, was late for the hundred-yard dash and stripped down to his BVD's and lined up in the starting blocks. He won the race, confirming his reputation as the fastest runner in northern Missouri.

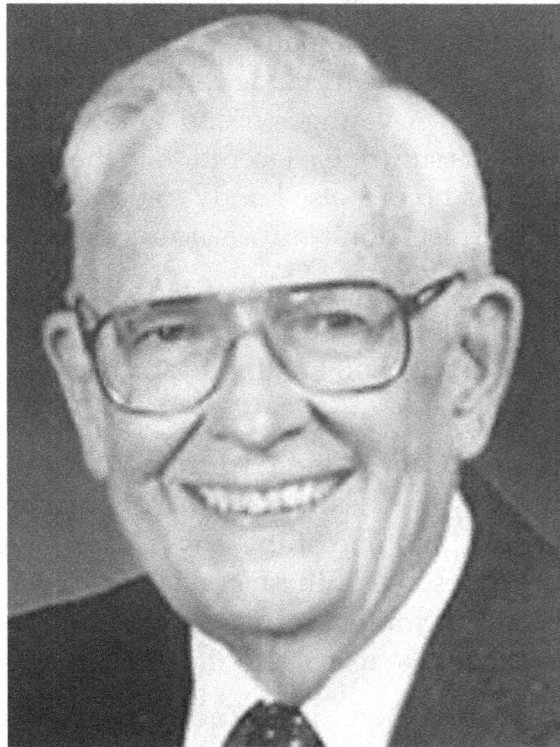

Lou Lambiotte (1920-2017) (Photo from Physicians and Medicine: Crawford and Sebastian Counties 1817-1976, by Amelia Martin, 1976)

I was fortunate to be introduced to Lou Lambiotte and have dinner with him and his wife Connie at Emmy's shortly after our family arrived in Fort Smith, and he proved to be a good friend, supportive to his younger colleague, from then on. As the only Fellow of the American College of Physicians in Fort Smith, he sponsored my application for fellowship, and we frequently saw each other at ACP meetings. His credentials were impeccable: A native of Fort Smith, he graduated from Fort Smith public schools and, in 1942, from the University of Arkansas where he was Phi Beta Kappa. He then graduated cum laude from Washington University in St. Louis, where he was in Alpha Omega Alpha, the medical scholastic honor society. He was selected for a coveted internship at Barnes Hospital, where he met Connie Gallentine, a nurse who became his wife; and he served as a Captain in the Medical Corps of the U.S. Army from 1946 to 1948. After his military duty at the Veterans Hospital in North Little Rock, he did his residency in internal medicine at the University of Utah from 1948 to 1951. He published a paper on tuberculosis in psychotic patients in 1949, and he joined Holt-Krock Clinic in 1951.

He seemed to be the perpetual chairman of the internal medicine section at Sparks, and he set a high standard of professionalism in his personal practice; I thought of him as my senior resident whenever I made rounds at Sparks (where we usually saw each other late at night). A younger friend who was an internist at Sparks, David Staggs, told me he was suturing a laceration in the Sparks Emergency Room one time, because there was no one else handy to do it, when he felt a tap on his shoulder. It was Lou. "Internists don't suture lacerations."

He was a quiet man, fastidious in writing progress notes and attentive to his patients. With no medical school in Fort Smith at that time, there were no local academic professors of medicine. Lou Lambiotte and Ken Thompson were my role models.

Many soldiers came through Camp Chaffee during World War II, and quite a few of them made Fort Smith their home after the war, often after marrying Fort Smith girls. Some were physicians, and one of these was Zach Hornberger, who did all the above, also documenting some of these crucial life experiences in a diary. His son Robert Hornberger, a Fort Smith attorney, has kept these firsthand fragments, and they provide details that take us back to the time and place.

The Hornberger family lived in Nebraska. Zach's memoir relates that one of his grandfathers was a physician who moved from Pennsylvania to Nebraska; the other, an itinerant minister and educator. His father was a banker during the time of the Great Depression, which led to some job changes and relocations of the family. Zach had rickets as a child and grew up on a buttermilk diet. He describes himself as having been the "fat boy in the neighborhood," but in high school he did play football. When the family moved to California he attended the University of Southern California, but the family returned to Omaha where he attended medical school at the University of Nebraska, commuting daily from home. He was fourth in his class and was named to the honor society Alpha Omega Alpha. Upon receiving his MD, he enlisted in the Medical Corps as a lieutenant and was granted a one-year deferment for internship, which he served at Columbia Hospital in Milwaukee. He began his military duty in July 1943, spending six weeks at Carlisle Barracks, Pennsylvania, before being sent to Camp Chaffee.

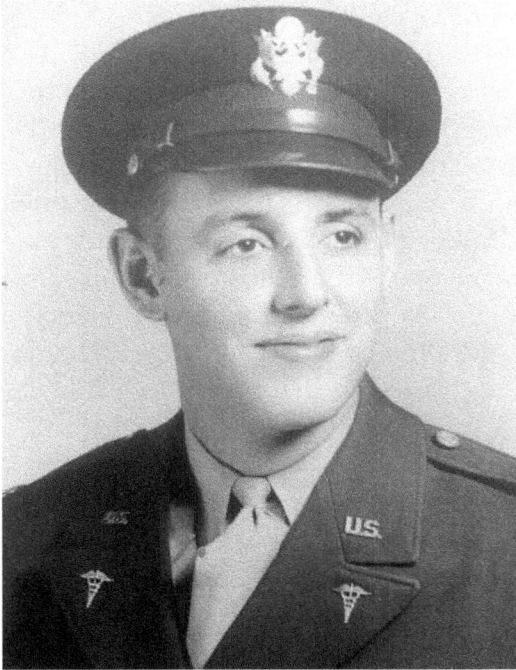

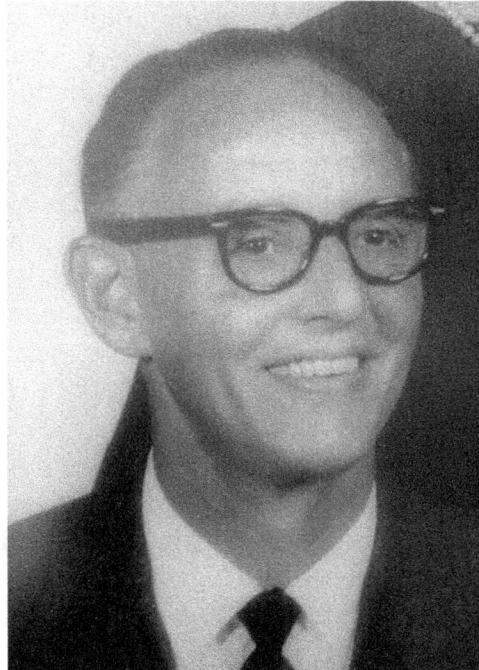

Zach Hornberger (1918-2000) (Photos courtesy of Robert Hornberger)

These selected diary entries provide pertinent details about life in Fort Smith and, graphically, the firsthand observations of the life of an army medic in the war:

> Hardscrabble Country Club had a deal where we could use the club for five dollars a month, which we did. On one occasion we met Betty Porter (Warner now) and Ed Bedwell, and they told me to call Nancy Eads if we wanted to meet some nice people. This I did, and she agreed to have Bruce [Graham] and me come into her house to meet her and the friend, the sister of the man Nancy was pinned to. It was love at first sight for me, and after several dates I proposed, and she accepted in late October 1943. [What happened to the man Nancy was pinned to?] She and her mother and I drove all night to Omaha in November to meet my family and announce our engagement. There was gas rationing, and we didn't

115

have enough stamps, but because I was in uniform, many people gave us gas without stamps. I was billeted in a tarpaper shack in the 16th Division—it was a cold winter—and after we were engaged, the Eads let me sleep in their guestroom on nights when I was not on duty.

[In another note, Zach listed Nancy's family] Nancy's paternal grandfather was Charles B. Eads, a cofounder of Eads Brothers Furniture Company in Fort Smith. Her paternal grandmother was Elizabeth Barnes Eads. Her maternal grandfather was William Ben Cravens who was an attorney and served in Congress for many years. Her maternal grandmother was Caroline Dye Cravens.

Nancy and I were married on January 7, 1944, a Friday at six PM, in the Eads home at 130 Sweet St., during a huge snowstorm (14 inches total). We tried to leave for Hot Springs for our honeymoon, but the snow was so bad that we had to turn back, and we spent the night in the Ward Hotel. Missy Armstrong (age 10) was Nancy's attendant, and my brother John was my best man. John sang the song "To You," which Mother had written. Bill Eads, Jr. was home from Culver, and he and Bud Jackson, Jim Holder, and some others did their best to drink all the champagne in Sebastian County that night. At three AM that night Nancy was hungry, so I went across the street to the Wide-Awake Café to get a ham sandwich. Bill Jr. and several of my army buddies were there and I took a real ribbing for a long time.

Nancy and I had rented a small house at 1104 S. 26th St. from the Ralph Motts, so we started to move in the day after the wedding. We finally got out of town —had a hair-raising trip to Hot Springs on Sunday but had to come home two days later because Nancy's dog Tillie wouldn't eat or drink. We enjoyed having our own home, and I commuted to Chaffee daily for work.

Zach was sent to Camp Butner in March 1944, to the 35th Infantry Division, and from there to Europe.

We were put on a troop ship and left the USA on May 1st, 1944. We had a very rough crossing in a huge convoy—lost several ships to German Subs—and arrived at Southampton, England. We later landed on Omaha Beach on July 7th—had to wade through waist-deep water for one hundred or more yards to the beach—moved up steep bluffs into a bivouac area, and lots of gunfire and artillery, but didn't know how far away it was—artillery duel tonight lasted thirty minutes—everyone in foxholes—a strange, sobering, and frightening experience at night.

July 19—our first German air raid—lots of bombs ahead – flares everywhere – scared us good.

July 22—artillery duel tonight lasted 30 minutes—everyone in foxholes

July 25—beautiful day—constant cover of B-17 and P-47 overhead flying forts and Libs who dropped tons of bombs saw one Lib go down in flames from flack followed by P-38s and P-51s bombing and strafing.

July 27—German planes bombed and strafed after 2300 hours—scared hell out of all of us.

July 28—moved ahead today. Another German air raid—were in foxholes but brought in casualties so had to get out and work on them with no protection. Bomb destroyed one of our ambulances. One of our men went berserk tonight—had a hard time controlling and evacuating him.

July 31, 1944 —air raids by Germans every night— new area yesterday—worked until one AM on casualties. Hot today.

August 6—moved out of combat August 4 into rest area. French farm next to us —traded soap for eggs and a shot of Calvados (WOW), slept up against hedgerow—won't sleep out of foxhole again—heavy air raid.

August 11-13—battle of Mortain —heavy casualties not so many air raids

August 13-14—moved in convoy all night had abscessed tooth pulled at Evac hospital.

August 15—left Le Mans during night—traveled all night and most of day to Châteaudun front—weather hot—French people gave us great welcome—work very heavy—so tired can hardly see.

August 17—closer to town—no casualties —but fruit and champagne

August 19—move to Janville—heavy rain which soaked me in tent.

August 20—dried clothes all day—no work

August 27—chills & fever—bad throat food situation is awful.

August 28—throat OK with aspirin and sulfa

August 29—rain all day moved into French château out of town.

August 30—running again—French farmer gave us a roasted goose potatoes eggs tomatoes and Calvados for cigarettes and chocolate.

September 3—Transferred to A company with Fred Webster—set up in French infirmary—Fred and I celebrated with too much champagne— spent morning treating Sir Malcolm Campbell's wife for overdose of sleeping pills—spent afternoon in city of Troyes—Lots of champagne and cognac around.

September 11—close to Michelle River instrument factory—our troops were trapped during night trying to cross river—almost wiped out second Battalion. Casualties very heavy—worked all night and all day—Fred Webster wounded last night but refused evacuation—OK.

September 15—moved across river last night and in the city of Nancy today—mobbed by civilians—rescued American prisoners—shut up in large hospital—baths, white sheets on beds, and dinner with local MDs

September 17—moved across Canal—put up in private homes—saw French woman collaborator severely beaten.

November 9—rainy and miserable set up in good building in town of Betancourt outside of Nancy. I have a comfortable setup casualties light Air Force blew up dam near here—flood all around us. Several shows here—Marlene Dietrich was on

November 10—first snowfall—moved to Contieres—town a wreck.

November 13—worst day yet—220 casualties from eight AM to six AM

Brought in a soldier for me to pronounce dead—felt faint pulse in neck, so treated with adrenaline, caffeine, and plasma, and he woke up and talked to us before they evacuated him. Great feeling!

November 15—call—lots of snow—I have cold, cough, and backache.

December 7—Germans helped us celebrate Pearl Harbor Day with thirty rounds of artillery very close by—three hits on our building and knocked out two ambulances and a truck.

December 9—shells within a block of us—snipers in town—shooting at medics—staying inside.

December 16—moved again—told I am to be transferred into first battalion aid station—feel lousy—eating very poorly—usually only one meal a day.

December 17—rainy and miserable—with aid station temporary—terrible place to try to work—moved offline yesterday back to Putelange and clearing company—have had movies, shows, radios etc.

December 23—left Putelange at four AM—extremely cold—to Metz where they say we will stay.

December 25, 1944—Christmas day in Metz—great dinner—no work

December 26—left Metz six AM—to near Arion north of Luxembourg—very cold

December 27—moved to Warnach in Belgium—rode jeep nine hours—very cold.

December 30—Germans firing rockets (screaming mimis) at us—weird sound.

December 31—blizzard last night—casualties heavy—German tanks only 500 yards from us—had to abandon aid station—walked in blizzard from five PM to midnight back to Warnach—horrible we didn't have a password and were afraid we would be shot by our own men!

January 1, 1945—great turkey dinner—I moved my half of the company into Bastogne—three ambulances and one jeep—third ambulance got a direct hit by German artillery—killed two of our men and destroyed vehicle—set up in large room on first floor in the basement—tried to sleep on second floor in a bed, but too much shelling and too scared to stay.

January 2—still in Bastogne in same set up—casualties light—incoming and outgoing artillery unbelievable—Germans have closed access to Bastogne—no one really knows we are here. Blew roof off buildings next to us—cold and miserable weather. Barrages daily and constant—engineers found a buried wine cellar full of really good wine – I got a case of red and of white. Lots of P-47's overhead

January 24—we left Bastogne today—to Trois Verges—bitterly cold with lots of snow and no heat.

January 25—no casualties—army still pushing Germans back—moved back to Rumlange in schoolhouse—still away from our 35th Division. Bored and lonesome—nothing to do.

February 1—moved through Bastogne, Marche, Liège, to Maastricht, and back with 35th Division in monastery—great party to welcome us.

February 3—visited 41st Evacuation hospital. What a set up—went to Aachen Germany—tremendous destruction—evening in Maastricht at USO.

February 10—moved back to Gangelt, Germany—Germans blew up a dam and flooded area close to us.

February 13—to Maastricht—tub bath—officers PX here—movies

February 17—lots of movies last three days. No work—back to Geilenkirchen

February 19—spent day in Brussels just sightseeing—too expensive to buy anything. Stayed here until February 26

March 7, 1945—moved into civilian hospital—went with Fred Webster and driver to small town on Rhine River (Rhineberg—can't find on map) found a good spot in a brewery for station—got caught in mortar barrage on corner while walking back to jeep—I was hit in the left arm and side—rolled into a ditch until the barrage was over—bleeding bad—ran into a nearby house—G.I. used his belt to put a tourniquet on my arm, or I would've probably bled to death. Driver not hit—Fred hit in left arm and leg—ambulance from company came and took us through our clearing station to the 100th Evac hospital. Doctors there wanted to amputate my arm because the brachial artery had been severed and the nerves damaged. I talked them out of the amputation, and instead they kept me five days and gave me stellate ganglion blocks every four to five hours (very painful).

March 13—evacuated to the shore 32nd General Hospital in Aachen

March 14—hospital train to Liège—to holding hospital—then flown from Liège to England and the 130th Station hospital. My arm was still viable but completely paralyzed.

March 17—made ambulatory and moved to 94th General Hospital. Extremely weak

March 19—surgical closure of wounds

(This is the end of my diary.)

I don't remember how long I stayed in England but was then put on a hospital ship (converted Liberty ship) with many other casualties and transported to Camp Kilburn, New Jersey. Very rough stormy crossing, and I was extremely seasick all the way.

Was put on a hospital train at Kilmer—was ambulatory so I was put in charge of my car—we stopped briefly in Omaha, and I got to see Mom and Dad. Went on to Ogden, Utah. and then to Bushnell General Hospital in Brigham City, Utah. Nancy and her dad drove our old 1940 Ford to Ogden where I met them—I had on the same suit of wool OD clothes I had been wearing since leaving England. Nancy's dad left immediately by train for home. Nancy and I first had a room with no bath in an attic—really bad set up. We soon moved to a much better room on the second floor of a dentist's home—shared a bath with the Mazzantis from Lake Village but had no (**end of text**)

He was discharged as a captain.

Dr. Hornberger had planned to practice obstetrics and gynecology, but his injury to his left arm and hand left him with a loss of dexterity that led him to change to general practice, later restricting his practice to internal medicine. He and Nancy moved to Milwaukee where he practiced until 1950 when Dr. Tom Foltz persuaded him to return to Fort Smith where he joined Drs. Foltz and Drs. Marlin and Arthur Hoge. He later established an internal medicine clinic with Drs. Hugh Lewing, Larry Price, and Paul Schwarz.

Dr. Hornberger was a central figure in Fort Smith medicine, organizing a high-quality internal medicine clinic and serving as the first medical director of Sparks Regional Medical Center after his retirement from private practice. Dr. Price, who joined him in practice in 1969, recalls him as one who engaged readily with his patients, making them feel comfortable as he efficiently filled out his record of the office visit, listing the patient's history in the upper left quadrant of his note, physical examination findings in the upper right, lab data and diagnosis in the lower left, and medications and follow-up in the lower right quadrant.

Dr. Hornberger's son Bob recalls two stories that give a glimpse of the house call era. When he arrived at the home of one elderly woman who occasionally called, he would find a trail of dollar bills leading from the front door to her bedroom where she was waiting to see him. That was his fee. On another occasion he was called to an address that turned out to be a vacant lot, where a rowdy group of young men were waiting to steal his medical bag for drugs. He got away, but that was his last house call.

He became Director of Medical Education at Sparks, a position which he largely created, in 1975.

"Son, when you go into a patient's room, sit down, cross your legs, and take your time; and even if you're just there for five minutes, they'll think it's a half hour.

Speak to everybody in the room; and before you leave, be sure to ask if there are any more questions." How many young doctors get this kind of instruction from their father? Much less learn how to do a stellate ganglion block? This was R.C. Goodman, the first anesthesiologist to practice in Fort Smith, speaking to his son, a young plastic surgeon, who now refers to his father as "the kindest, humblest, most caring person I've known." OK, knock off a few points for filial bias; that still leaves a testimonial that any father would covet.

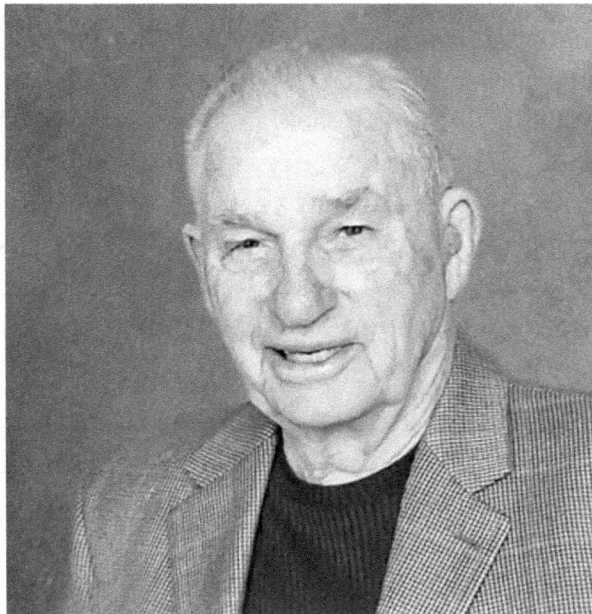

R.C. Goodman (1920-2014) (Photo courtesy of Dr, Cole Goodman)

R.C. Goodman grew up in rural southwestern Arkansas to parents who had eighth and sixth grade educations. (That was his name, by the way. "R.C." on the birth certificate, given the name Raymond Cole Goodman by an employer of the young lad who said he had to have a first name and a middle name and that he would give them to him. And so that's where R.C.'s son Cole got his name.) He studied business administration at Magnolia A & M (now Southern State University) and played guard on the football team. His National Guard unit was mobilized in December 1940, and he spent two years in Nome, Alaska, then returned to the States for officers' training.

Among 15,000 troops crossing the ocean to England on the Queen Mary, Goodman spent one day as escort to Winston Churchill and his wife Clemmie. Churchill gave him two cigars, one to use when he got to France and one for when he crossed the Rhine into Germany. He was in Belgium for the Battle of the Bulge, which was fought in bitter cold. His battle experiences were traumatic, including crossing a mine-laden field, with only fourteen of forty-one soldiers surviving the ordeal. He never participated in Fourth of July celebrations after he got home, because the fireworks reminded him too much of such experiences as this. It was in watching the victims of the war, whom he could do nothing significant to help, that he decided to go to medical school after he returned from the war.

First, he had to complete his pre-med requirements, which he did at the University of Arkansas. Then he got his MD at UAMS in Little Rock and became one of the earliest residents in anesthesiology at Parkland Hospital in Dallas. He joined Holt-Krock Clinic in 1955, where he was the only anesthesiologist in the area for several years. His particular interest was in management of chronic pain, and he began the regular practice of pain management in 1986 at Sparks. A center for this purpose was dedicated in 1991, named the R.C. Goodman Institute of Pain Management in his honor. He retired at age seventy-two and died in his ninety-fourth year.

Dr. Marlin B. Hoge, who died in 2017 at the age of one hundred three, was a formidable figure in Fort Smith medicine. Indeed, it was said that when he and his father, Dr. Arthur Hoge (1887–1954), stepped off the elevator at one of the floors of St. Edward Hospital, the nurses would say to one another, in the irreverent humor that one might sometimes find in a Catholic hospital, "Here comes the Lord God Almighty and Little Baby Jesus." Arthur Hoge was born in Nebraska but grew up in Mena. He graduated from Tulane, interned at Touro Infirmary in New Orleans, spent a year in Nicaragua, and began practice in Fort Smith in 1911. Their house was on Free Ferry, and Marlin told me about riding his horse to Fort Smith High School on one occasion, a form of transportation that the school did not approve of. Marlin recalled going with his father to Ozark to operate in the kitchen of a rural farmhouse in the 1920s.

Marlin told me the story of his own appendectomy several times in his later years, and I've heard similar versions of the same story from some of his other younger friends. As a medical student, Marlin was at home in Fort Smith when he developed appendicitis. His father told him that there was no anesthesiologist available, but that he could perform the appendectomy without general anesthesia. He did so, and Marlin was out of the hospital the next day. Dr. Hoge thought that since that operation went so well with such a rapid recovery that he could do it on the next patient. But that patient screamed and jumped around on the table so much that he quickly had to abandon the attempt.

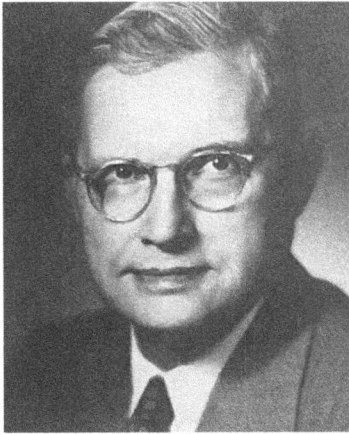

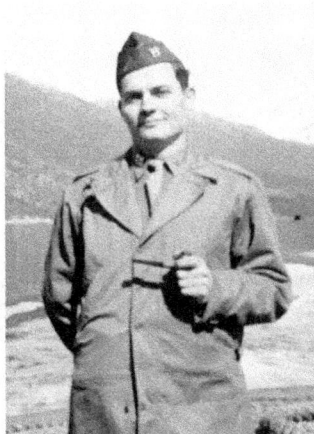

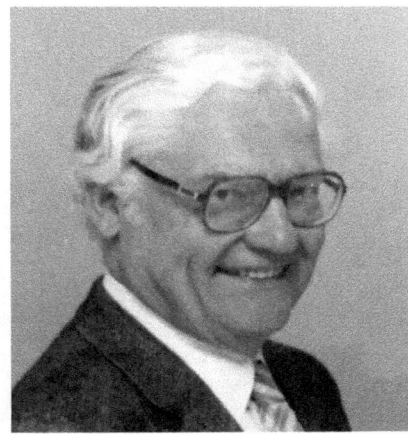

Arthur Hoge (1887-1954) (photo from Physicians and Medicine: Crawford and Sebastian Counties 1817-1976, by Amelia Martin, 1976)

Marlin B. Hoge (1914-2017), during World War II and after retirement (Photos from Dignity Memorial obituary)

Dr. William E. "Bill" Knight began the orthopedic department at Holt-Krock Clinic in 1948 after a training history that was hardly traditional. He was born and raised in New Brunswick, Canada, then attended the Massachusetts College of Osteopathy in Boston and the Kirksville College of Osteopathy and Surgery in Missouri, graduating with a DO degree in 1932. After an internship in Los Angeles, he practiced osteopathy in Maine. He moved to Madill, Oklahoma, in 1935 to escape the Maine winters; but then in 1937 he decided to enter medical school and enrolled in the Murray State School of Agriculture while still practicing as an osteopath. He received his BS degree from Southeastern State College in Durant, Oklahoma, and his MD degree in 1943 from the University of Oklahoma School of Medicine. After an internship and one year of residency in orthopedics in Oklahoma City, he served in the U.S. Army in Puerto Rico from 1945 to 1947—part time as a ship's doctor. He then completed his orthopedic residency at St. Anthony Hospital and the McBride Bone and Joint Hospital in Oklahoma City. He moved to Fort Smith as Holt-Krock Clinic's first orthopedist in 1948.

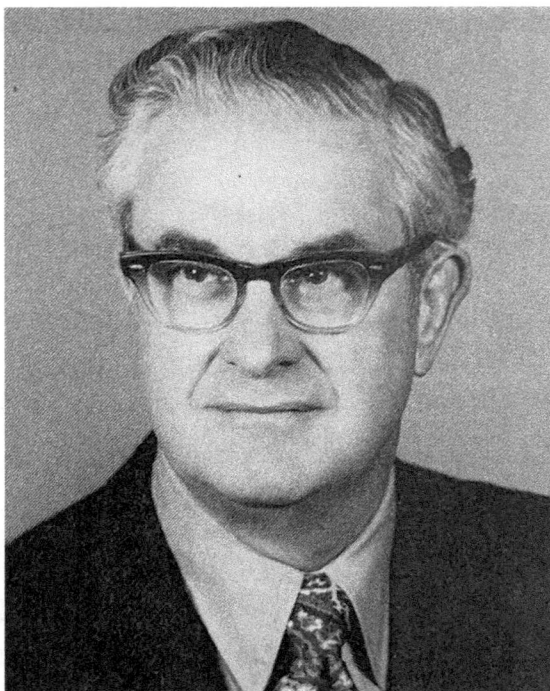

William E. Knight (199-2003) (Photo from Physicians and Medicine: Crawford and Sebastian Counties 1817-1976, by Amelia Martin, 1976)

Under Dr. Knight's leadership, the Holt-Krock orthopedic department attracted skilled surgeons who set a high standard of practice in the area. Among his other professional associations, he founded and served as president of the Arkansas Orthopedic Society. In 1949 he also founded the Orthopedic Letters Club, an international organization that did volunteer service in Israel, Jordan, and other countries. In this connection he worked eight weeks in Israel and Jordan in 1960. The work of this organization was later taken over and continued by Care-Medico. He was a perfectionist in all he did, especially in the operating room, and a former associate administrator of St. Edward recalls that when he first started in the 1970s, he was summoned to the operating room by one of the nuns who said that Dr. Knight was displeased and had thrown an instrument.

I knew him mostly as a fellow amateur photographer and a good friend in his retirement years, who won prizes in Fort Smith Art Center competitions with his travel photography. I still recall his compliment of my work: "One thing about your pictures: they're sharp." This was high praise from someone who was sharp in all he did. He was better known as a sailor, serving as commodore of the Central States Sailing Association and locally as president of the Fort Smith Sailing Club.

The Fort Smith Regional Art Museum (RAM) owns a large collection of Boehm porcelain bird sculpture which it displays in the Dr. William E. Knight Porcelain Gallery, a major part of the museum's permanent gallery, according to the museum website. Bill and his wife Chancey started this collection with a donation of eleven pieces from their personal collection in 1975, later adding more pieces for a total of seventy-seven.

Bill and Chancey retired to Blaine, Washington, in the 1990s. He died in 2003 at the age of ninety-four.

Perhaps one marker of professionalism in doctors is what they look like at two a.m. (and how they act). Dr. Thomas P. Foltz (1909-1974) set a high standard in this regard. More than one colleague who saw him in the night reports that when he was called to the hospital, he always appeared with suit and tie, neatly pressed, perhaps a vest, and shoes shined, before changing to scrubs if surgery was indicated. Dr. Foltz was a second-generation Fort Smith physician, son of Dr. James Arthur Foltz, who came to Fort Smith with his parents in 1881 when he was three years old. He was a sergeant in the U.S. Army during the Spanish-American War, graduated from Tulane University School of Medicine as class president and valedictorian, did postgraduate work at Harvard, and trained in surgery at hospitals in New York. He practiced medicine and surgery in Fort Smith until his death in 1937, serving on the school board and earning the following eulogy from editor C.F. Byrns: "His was a radiant personality, combining rare ability in his profession with a deep love of beauty and personal charm."

Back to Dr. Tommy Foltz: Like his father, he was president of his graduating class at Tulane School of Medicine. He trained at Touro Infirmary in New Orleans and began his practice in Fort Smith with his father in 1936. Entering the U.S. Navy in 1942, he served in the Naval Medical Corps in the Southwest Pacific. After the war he was assigned to the naval induction center in Little Rock, and he was a captain at the time of his discharge from the navy in 1945. He took a preceptorship under a Navy friend in Beverly Hills, California, and then he returned to practice in Fort Smith. In addition to his practice of surgery, he served on the school board, board of trustees of Sparks, and on the board of Arkansas Blue Cross and Blue Shield. He and his wife Eleanor Albers had two sons, Thomas Foltz Jr. (1937-2020) and Judge Harry Foltz (born 1939). Dr. Foltz retired in 1969 and died in 1974.

A doctor who was recognized in the community for continued service after retirement was Dr. Art Martin, who founded the Fort Smith Trolley Museum in 1985, after he and his wife Amelia had been working on it since 1979. It now has one and a half miles of track in downtown Fort Smith, four of Fort Smith's fifty-eight trolley cars, and several railroad cars. Dr. Martin grew up in Greenwood, was Alpha Omega Alpha at the University of Arkansas School of Medicine, where he graduated sixth in his class, and interned at Baptist Hospital in Little Rock. He received the Bronze Star for his service in the European Theater in World War II, where he was a battalion surgeon and was discharged in 1945 as a Captain. He was in the internal medicine department of Holt-Krock Clinic until 1983 and subsequently served as medical director of the Methodist Nursing Home until 2003, when he retired at age eighty-six. He continued to go to the trolley museum on Saturdays until a month before he died at age ninety-five.

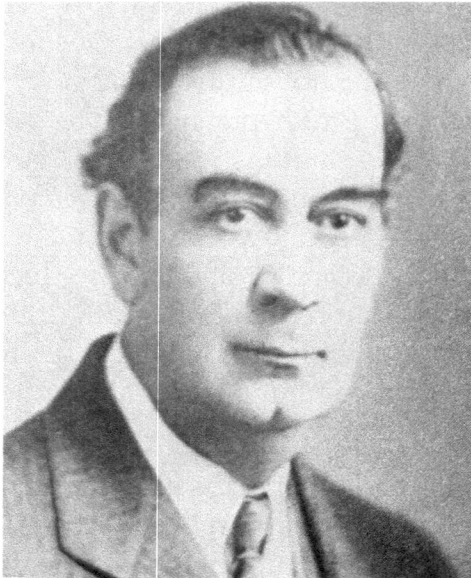

James A. Foltz (1878-1937)   *Thomas P. Foltz (1909-1974)*
(Photos courtesy of Harry Foltz)

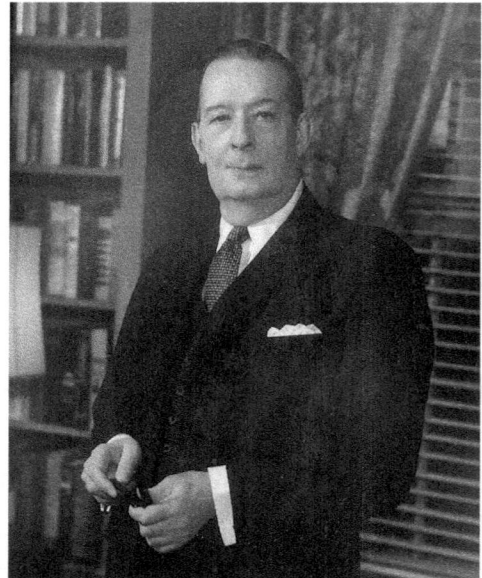

As mentioned, these doctors are only representatives of those who practiced in Fort Smith in mid-twentieth century. All are now deceased. They interrupted their personal and professional lives to do things they didn't particularly want to do, because it had to be done. Their experiences were perilous and often quite unpleasant, and some of their companions did not survive. They returned battle-scarred, and they practiced medicine with the same sense of duty that had served them well in war. Their high level of competence did indeed create a medical renaissance and provided high quality medical care to their community, and they left a high standard of performance for their successors.

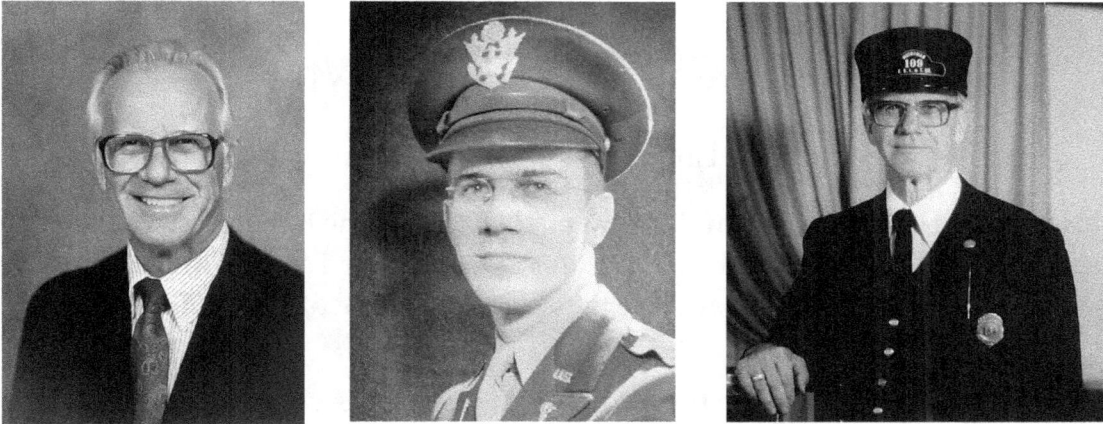

Art B. Martin (1917-2013) in military uniform and as trolley car conductor (Photos courtesy of Dignity Memorial obituary

One of those who served his country in wartime returned to Fort Smith to play a role in another facet of medical care that was just beginning to be revolutionized: the social changes that convulsed the nation in the 1960s and developed into an ongoing struggle for equal opportunities and equal rights. As we will see in the next chapter, Fort Smith was one of many communities coping with these issues; and in Fort Smith, the agent of change was Dr. Harry P. McDonald.

He Knew Who He Was

Reflections on the Life and Mission of Harry P. McDonald

Good stories take on a life of their own. The story of the integration of the Boston Store Tea Room in Fort Smith is one of these; it's too good a story to hold still. Here is the story, which I heard several times, as told by one of Harry McDonald's old friends:

It was a quiet morning at the Boston Store on Garrison Avenue. This was 1963; sit-ins had begun in Greensboro, North Carolina, in 1960, and Little Rock had experienced its season of sit-ins in November 1962. Dr. Harry McDonald and a group of other members of the National Association for the Advancement of Colored People (NAACP) walked into the Boston Store and on to the Tea Room, where they told the hostess they had come to integrate the Tea Room.

"Oh, Dr. McDonald. Wait just a minute, and I'll go get Mr. Ney."

McDonald and Jerome Ney, owner of the Boston Store, had sat in on several meetings to plan for integration of business places in Fort Smith, and the group waited. But when Mr. Ney appeared, it was the younger Mr. Ney.

"Dr. McDonald, this is my first day at work, and my father is out today. Could you come back and integrate the Tea Room on another day when my father is here?"

The group departed. And the Tea Room was integrated—but not that day. [1] Harry McDonald and Jerome Ney had both been among those appointed by Mayor Robert Brooksher to the Mayor's Committee on Race Relations to address the issue of desegregation of lunch counters. [2]

After this story appeared in the paper I wrote for the *Journal of the Fort Smith Historical Society*, I received a call from the only participant in this story who is still living: Randy Ney in Beaumont, Texas, where he has lived for several decades. "Nobody will ever know except you and me, but I want to get the facts straight. It was in the early '60s, and Harry came to the store one time and wanted to talk to my dad. He wasn't available, so Harry came to my office. I was relatively new on the job."

"My wife and I have been buying our clothes in your store for over fifteen years."

"Yes sir, I know that."

"I buy my Hickey Freeman suits here."

"Yes, sir, I know."

"My wife buys the finest dresses here." (Randy mentioned a couple of brand names that I don't remember.)

"Yes, sir, I know."

"But we can't eat in your tearoom. Can we avoid a sit-in?"

"I told him I'd have to talk to my dad. Dad and I agreed that we had to be in the forefront of integrating our store."

"So, I went back to Dr. McDonald. I told him our employees have to get used to the idea. And our loyal customers had to get used to it. I suggested that he and Mrs. McDonald come to the Tea Room in the middle of the afternoon some time when it's not too busy. We would serve them. Then the next time come a little earlier in the afternoon. After three or four visits they might come at noon. Dad and I could join them at the table."

"He agreed, and that's what we did." [3]

This was Harry McDonald's style (and Jerome Ney's style). According to his son Palmer McDonald, "He worked behind the scenes, but he was persistent." He was president of the Fort Smith chapter of the NAACP from 1960 to 1970. During this time there were so many members that they had to meet in the Ninth Street Baptist Church, [4] and several major changes occurred during this decade. Perhaps the most memorable of these was the integration of Northside High School, accomplished after the NAACP sued the Fort Smith School Board in the Sebastian County Circuit Court in 1963. The NAACP lost in the Circuit Court and appealed to the Eighth Circuit Court of Appeals and lost again. The United States Supreme Court overturned the two lower court rulings in December 1965, and ordered the Fort Smith School District to desegregate its senior high schools.

The court issued its ruling without hearing oral arguments, on a 5-4 vote, saying, "Petitioners are entitled to immediate relief. We have emphasized that delays in desegregating public school systems are no longer tolerable." At this time Fort Smith had desegregated the first nine grades, following a stairstep plan begun in 1957 with the first grade. Lincoln High School, the school for African Americans, had a faculty that included well-educated, well-trained teachers; but Lincoln only offered thirty-four different courses, compared to sixty-four at Northside. And because of the ruling, the first two African American students graduated from Northside in 1966. [5]

Dr. McDonald began his practice of medicine in Fort Smith in 1949 and retired in 1990. He was born in 1923 in Sumter, South Carolina, a city begun as a plantation settlement near the geographic center of South Carolina. His father worked for the railway postal system, taught at Claflin College, and was president of the Sumter chapter of the NAACP. His mother taught music. His paternal grandfather, Robert John Palmer, Sr., served in the South Carolina House of Representatives from 1876 to 1878 during the last years of Reconstruction after the Civil War.

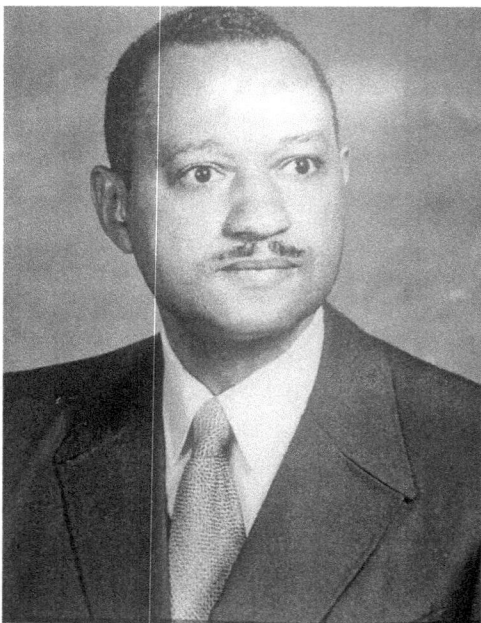

Harry McDonald (Photo courtesy of Pebley Center, UAFS)

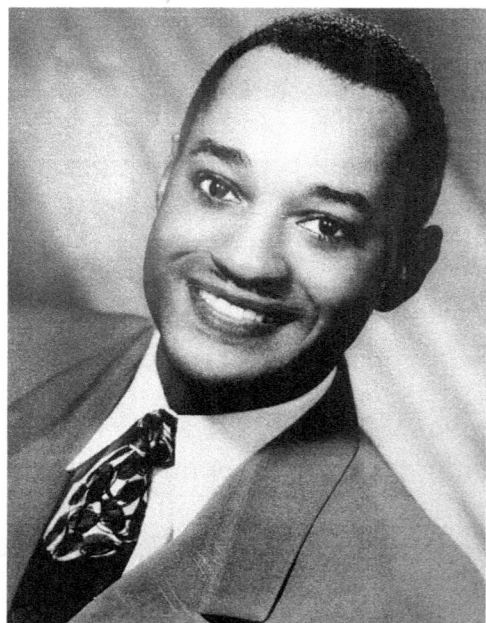

Young Harry McDonald (Photo courtesy of Pebley Center, UAFS)

Status, family, and role in life played a significant part in African-American society in the South, especially in cities such as Atlanta, but also in smaller communities. Whatever this distinction was called—aristocracy, meritocracy, or classes such as upper middle class—it was a reality; and in Sumter, a city of 40,000 where half the population was black, education was a key factor in defining class status. Here Robert Palmer's descendants excelled. One of his sons, Edmund Perry Palmer, graduated from Claflin College and was the first of four generations in the funeral profession, owning and operating Palmer Chapel in Sumter. Edmund's son Bob, second in the family to operate the funeral home, was Harry's cousin and best friend. Bob's brother Jim Palmer was an internist in Atlanta and personal physician to Martin Luther King, Jr. [6] Another second cousin, Mary McCleod Bethune, was founder of Bethune-Cookman College. Harry and two of his brothers became physicians; his third brother was a dentist. And Harry, in turn, would not let any of his four children take out a loan for college education; he paid for it himself, and all four obtained advanced degrees. Harry did not retire until Maria, his youngest, had graduated from college. [7]

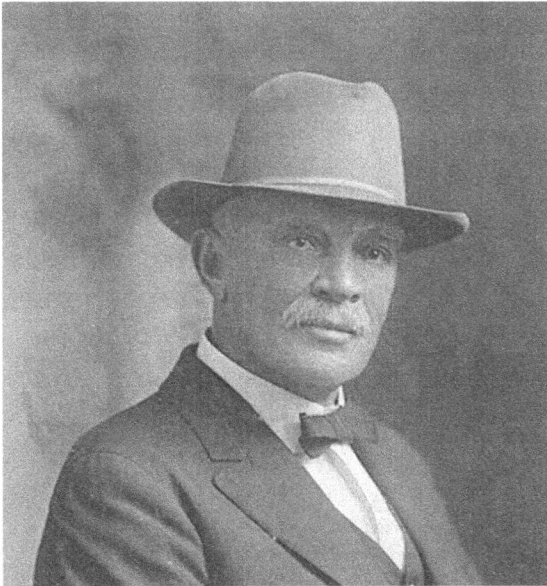

Robert John Palmer (1849-1928), Harry's maternal grandfather (Photo courtesy of Pebley Center, UAFS)

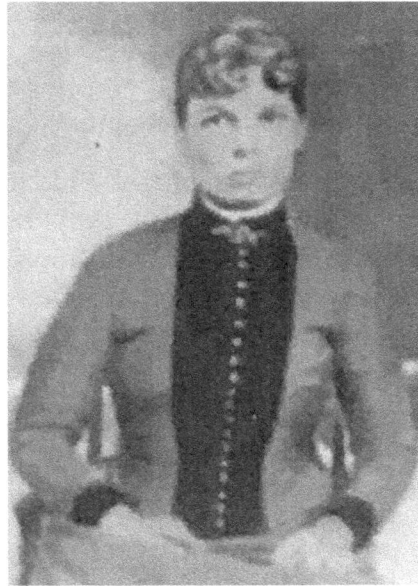

Harriet Elizabeth DesChamps McDonald (1845-1931), Harry's paternal grandmother (Pebley Center, UAFS)

Harry was valedictorian of his high school class, graduated from Morehouse College in Atlanta with honors (a few years before Martin Luther King, Jr. received his degree there), and then obtained his MD degree at Meharry Medical College. He did his internship at Harlem Hospital in New York and went on to Kansas City General Hospital for an internal medicine residency. He was planning to join his older brother Bruce in practice in Kansas City when Theodore Rutledge of Fort Smith came to Kansas City with the widow of Dr. Ernest Adolphus Dennard and persuaded him to come to Fort Smith in 1949. Dr. Dennard's death in 1948 had left Fort Smith without a black physician, and they were also eager to have a physician who could potentially become a leader in the NAACP. [8] Theodore Rutledge was especially persistent in recruiting Dr. McDonald, and Harry lived with Seth Rutledge, Theodore's uncle and president of NAACP in Fort Smith, for five years.

Harry found race relations in Fort Smith different from any in his previous experience, according to his son Palmer. There was a large black population in Sumter, segregation was an accepted way of life, and no one questioned it when Harry was growing up. Morehouse and Meharry were African American schools, and Harlem Hospital was in the African American section of New York. Kansas City had a significant middle-class black population in which Harry and his brother Bruce were comfortable. Fort Smith, on the other hand, had a minority black population of about ten percent, separate but far from equal. "Civil rights were behind in Fort Smith. Both blacks and whites were lethargic," Euba Winton, a Fort Smith matriarch, recalls.

After beginning his solo general practice in 1949, Harry was drafted into the Air Force in 1954. While driving his Buick from Fort Smith to San Francisco to begin his duty, he detoured to Williams, Arizona, to see the Grand Canyon. The motel manager there told him that there was no place for a black man to spend the night in Williams, but that he could find a place in Flagstaff. So, he drove back, arriving in Flagstaff two hours later at midnight, where he called the local sheriff and told him he was Captain Harry McDonald on his way to San Francisco and needed a place to stay for the night. The sheriff went to a motel and persuaded the owner to change his policy and allow Captain McDonald to stay for the night. [9]

Japan, where he was stationed from 1954 to 1956, was an eye-opening experience for Captain McDonald. There was no segregation; housing was integrated, and his roommate was white. And then after his discharge he came back to a segregated community, where his position in society was so different from what he had experienced in Japan that he resolved to join the struggle for equal rights. [10]

After they had known each other only six months, Harry and Margaret Bowling, a college professor from Columbia, South Carolina, were married in 1956. According to their son Palmer, it was an arranged marriage. Margaret is described as a brilliant woman. Unfortunately, however, it was a mismatch. They stayed together for thirteen years and had four gifted children—Jan, Anita, Palmer, and Maria—before separating and divorcing in 1970 when Palmer was nine and Maria was three years old. During the 1960s, however, they were a formidable team. Margaret was a "fireball," according to their daughter Maria. "She had passion, drive, and ambition, and she could not tolerate any hint of racism." His mother was more confrontational, Palmer says; his father was more reserved. "He was humble and fit himself in," Euba Winton recalls. "He came as an outsider, but he became an insider."

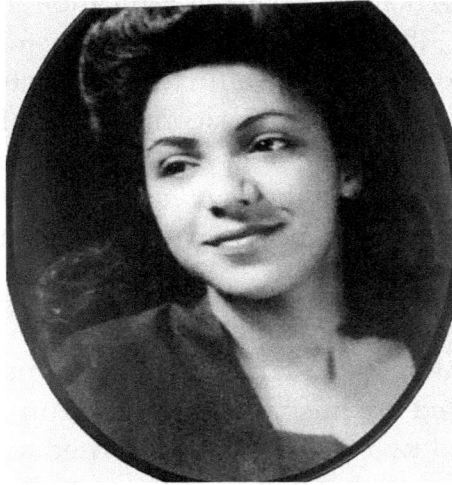

Margaret Bowling McDonald, Harry's wife until 1970 (Photo courtesy of Pebley Center, UAFS)

Harry married Ruby Bultman, a schoolteacher in Sumter, South Carolina, in 1976. This too was an arranged marriage, according to Maria. They were remote cousins, and Ruby's father owned a significant amount of property. Her personality was of the quieter sort, and their marriage was a source of stability to the family. The children initially lived with their mother after the divorce in 1970, but they began to return to live with their father, who gained custody five years after the divorce. One year later he married Ruby.

Harry was president of the Progressive Men's Club, composed mostly of black men and active in civil rights. He worked with Whirlpool, Gerber, and Dixie Cup to encourage employment and advancement of African Americans so that they could advance to supervision and middle management positions. He ran for the school board in the early 1960s. Election to the board was determined by a majority vote of citizens attending a town meeting at Northside High School. In an interview with the *Arkansas Democrat* in 1990, Dr. McDonald recalled that he had some five hundred supporters there, ready to vote for him. But minutes before the meeting was to begin, the superintendent of schools, Chris Corbin, postponed the meeting for half an hour. During that time, McDonald recalled, someone contacted the Knights of Columbus who were having a rally and bussed them to the meeting at Northside. "They emptied the bowling alley. Some of those people had bowling shoes and shirts on," he said. [**11,12**]

Though McDonald never served on the Fort Smith school board, Governor David Pryor named him to the Arkansas Board of Education in 1978, and he served for twelve years. Governor Bill Clinton appointed him to the Criminal Detention Facilities Review Committee for the Twelfth Judicial District in 1984. Advocacy for equality was never easy. "Life is full of conflict—it takes guts, patience, time, money, determination, and a certain degree of independence" to effect change, he said in an interview published in the *Southwest Times Record* at the time of his retirement. [**13**] For a quiet person, he could speak quite frankly.

He personally involved himself in integrating parks, movie theaters, skating rinks, and civic clubs. Although his encounter at the Boston Store was peaceful, the proprietor of a restaurant near St. Edward Hospital pulled a gun on him. The proprietor's wife persuaded her husband to put the gun away, but McDonald left. He went to the police, and two days later he returned to the same restaurant and was served. [**14**] When he took his daughter to the swimming pool at Creekmore Park, a city policeman pulled his pistol and turned him away. [**14**] "I always tried to be a good citizen of Fort Smith," he said later. "Even when I had to do battle, it was for the good of Fort Smith." [**15**]

Integration of movie theaters provided its own special circumstances. McDonald described sitting next to a white person in a theater, and there would be no notice in the dark theater until the light changed, and then the white person would move away. "People have come to realize that sitting next to a black person in a movie theater isn't going to do a white person any harm," he said. [**16**]

What motivated this quiet, pleasant man to push into segregated white society and pave the way for integration of the community? He himself said that it was because of the example of his father, who was very active in civil rights issues until his death in 1956. One also wonders if it was less difficult to shake things up as one who had come to Fort Smith as if it were a foreign mission field, where he was free of the baggage of having grown up in the city.

The Fort Smith city board of directors was about to name the Elm Grove Park on North Greenwood after Dr. McDonald in 1969, but he declined. This was a year after the assassination of Martin Luther King, Jr., and the youth chapter of the Fort Smith NAACP petitioned the city to name a street or park after King. The board first voted 3-2 for this proposal, with one abstention and one absentee; but four affirmative votes were required for passage. Then one of the directors, Rev. G.

Edward West, moved that the park be named for Dr. McDonald. The motion was seconded, but McDonald requested that his name be withdrawn, saying that if the directors wouldn't rename the park for as great a national figure as Dr. King, he wouldn't want it to bear his (McDonald's) name. After some discussion one of the directors, Bill Vines, said, "Your feelings against naming the park for a local man are apparently stronger than my feelings against naming it for Dr. King." Vines then moved that another vote be taken, and this time Vines joined another director, Harlin Daniels, in voting affirmatively, and the resolution renaming the park was approved. [17] And so with the naming of the park for the national champion of civil rights, the opportunity for the city to honor its own prophet passed by.

With all his civic involvement, McDonald's day (and night) job was practicing medicine as the only black physician in town. It was in this capacity that I knew him, and we sometimes found ourselves writing progress notes in a nursing station at St. Edward around nine to ten p.m., when the logical mindset for a fatigued physician is to finish rounds as quickly as possible and go home. Paradoxically, however, lengthy conversations sometimes occur at this time in a quiet and private setting, and Harry and I enjoyed talking shop, mostly. (I told his daughter Maria that his South Carolina speech background led him to call me "Tay-a-lah." "Oh, I can just hear him talking when you say that" Maria said.)

There were three hospitals in Fort Smith in 1949 when Dr. McDonald arrived: Sparks, St. Edward, and Twin City Hospital. (Twin City Hospital opened on 1717 Midland Boulevard in 1941 and provided health care to black citizens of Fort Smith; it was converted to a nursing home in 1964.) Twin City had no x-ray machines and no laboratory facilities. There was only one registered nurse, so patients were not permitted to stay overnight. [18] McDonald credited Father Deloney, of the St. John Catholic school for blacks on 1802 North Ninth Street, with helping him to gain privileges to practice at Crawford County Hospital when it was built by the county in 1951 and managed by the Sisters of St. Benedict. With a change in administration at St. Edward Hospital in Fort Smith, Dr. McDonald received admitting privileges there.

Black patients at St. Edward were on Ward 3B, where four rooms with four beds each were separated from the rest of the floor by a half door. Dr. McDonald became the first black physician on the Sparks staff five years later, in 1961. At that time black patients were admitted and were not placed in segregated areas.

Dr. McDonald became the first black member of the Sebastian County Medical Society and of the Arkansas Medical Society in the early 1960s. This wasn't so easy.

He recalled that when he first attended a meeting of the Sebastian County Medical Society, Dr. Everett Moulton was the only physician who would come sit by him and talk to him. The others would not. In later years, McDonald was elected president of the Sebastian County Medical Society. [19]

Dr. McDonald made house calls and delivered babies, and babies often come at night. He practiced alone and took his own calls, except on Wednesdays, when he took the afternoon off. Dr. Tommy Foltz was one of the few doctors who would see his patients for him; among the others who helped were Drs. Kemal Kutait and Ken Lilly. Dr. Foltz covered his calls when he was off and when he was on vacation. [9] That was two weeks a year, and his son Palmer says that his dad was so disciplined that he took off the same two weeks in the summer. During the first week he took the whole family to the annual meeting of the National Medical Association (founded in 1895 as an alternative to the whites-only American Medical Association). Palmer says that this was the only time he saw other black middle-class kids. During the second week Harry went alone to a hotel in the Bahamas—always the same hotel, and they knew him well there. "He went to the Caribbean because it was okay being a black there," Palmer explains. This was his vacation plan for thirty-five years—from the time he married until he retired.

Charlotte Tidwell, now a retired nurse who is founder and director of Antioch for Youth and Family food pantry, recalls that she was three years old in 1949 when Dr. McDonald came to Fort Smith. "My brother Nathaniel was eleven months older than I was, but he was always frail and sickly. My mother took him to Kansas City three times when she was pregnant with me, but they never made a diagnosis. Dr. McDonald made a diagnosis of leukemia. There was no cure, and he lived eleven more months, but at least we didn't have to make the trips to Kansas City."

"He was my idol, and because of him I was determined to be a nurse. He was the first black physician on the staff of St. Edward, and he persuaded the hospital nurse training program to accept black students." The first of these was Brenda Johnson, who gained admittance to the St. Edward Mercy Hospital School of Nursing in the fall of 1963 and graduated as the "Best All Around Student." She then moved to California, where she earned her Master of Public Health (MPH) degree at the University of California, Berkeley with a subsequent career at Aetna Health as a Team Captain for Western States. [20]

"Dr. McDonald taught me to get as much education as I could get," Charlotte Tidwell says. She was in the second class of African Americans at St. Edward, but she had to drop out when she married Lawrence Tidwell. She worked as a nurse's aide for three years, and by then Dr. McDonald had gained admission to the staff at Sparks Regional Hospital, and Sparks became the first nurses training program to accept married students. She was also the first black student there, but that was incidental, Tidwell says. She went on to receive several degrees and to become the director of medical-surgical nursing at Sparks.

Palmer and Maria both remember riding with their father to make night calls at the hospital and waiting in the car when he said he "would just be a minute." (Maria wondered if he was shooting the bull with me while she was waiting in the car.) Like many of the best-liked physicians, Dr. McDonald was often behind schedule because he took so much time with each patient. Some excellent cooks were among his patients, and Maria says she has learned to make the same Coca-Cola cake that Tabitha Hughes brought to their house at Christmas.

McDonald loved life and for that reason he hated death, Palmer says. Palmer recalls finding him in tears after one of his favorite patients died. Palmer says he never saw his father angry, but Euba Winton says that he had an even temper but could become very angry. Two of his great disappointments came when he attempted to buy a house in a white neighborhood and was blocked by action of the neighbors—once in a "doctors' circle" on the south side of town, [7] once in Eastwood just northeast of what is now the University of Arkansas Fort Smith campus. (When my family and I moved into Eastwood in 1969, we were told that Dr. McDonald had tried to buy a house on 58th Street, but the neighbors had bought the house to prevent integration of the neighborhood.) George McGill says that Dr. McDonald bought a six-lot property on 1823 North 30th Street and built a house on half of it. There are three houses on the rest of the property.

Euba Winton recalls that Mallalieu Methodist Church was a beehive of activity at that time, and that officers and soldiers from Fort Chaffee followed the McDonalds to Mallalieu, where McDonald was a lay leader and a trustee.

Governor Bill Clinton was the keynote speaker at the retirement dinner for McDonald in 1990, organized by Charlotte Tidwell. This was his farewell to Fort Smith. After a year in his hometown of Sumter, South Carolina, he moved to Fort Worth, Texas, to be near his daughter Anita.

Why did he leave? He told his son Palmer that he could never really retire and get away from the responsibilities and expectations that would overwhelm him unless he left town. After more than forty years on the front lines, he was exhausted. And although he could close his office, he couldn't have retired from the demands of being a prophet. A halo can be as heavy as a crown. Fort Smith had been his mission field. He loved the people, but like the cowboy in the western movies, sometimes the hero has to ride off into the sunset.

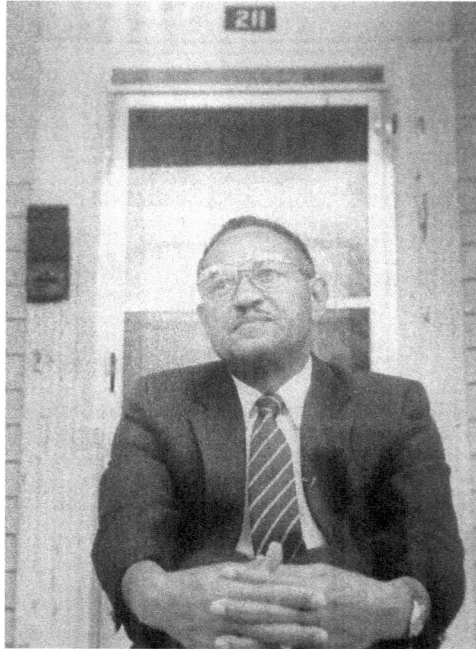

Harry at his boyhood home in Sumter, South Carolina (Photo courtesy of Pebley Center, UAFS)

There were other things he wanted to do. He wanted to play golf; the local courses had been inaccessible to blacks when he came to Fort Smith. Golf courses became integrated in due course, but this was one battle that McDonald left for someone else. He became a collector of art, especially the works of Sedrick Huckaby of Fort Worth. "His walls used to be covered by plaques," Palmer recalls. "Then they became covered by paintings."

I last saw Harry in 1995, when my family was vacationing at Hilton Head, South Carolina, where our custom was to attend services at St. Andrew-by-the-Sea Methodist Church. My son-in-law asked if a golf shirt would be all right for church on Sunday, and I told him not to worry, because we were sure not to see a soul we knew. During the service I spotted Harry McDonald. He was resplendent on this beautiful May morning, wearing the same white linen suit he had worn at his retirement dinner, and he had the same broad grin on his face. He introduced me to his cousin Bob, who lived in Sumter and had a condominium on Hilton Head. (Bob was Harry's lifelong best friend and died only a month later.) Harry said I was the first Fort Smith doctor he had seen since moving away, except Kemal Kutait, whom he had seen in Central Mall.

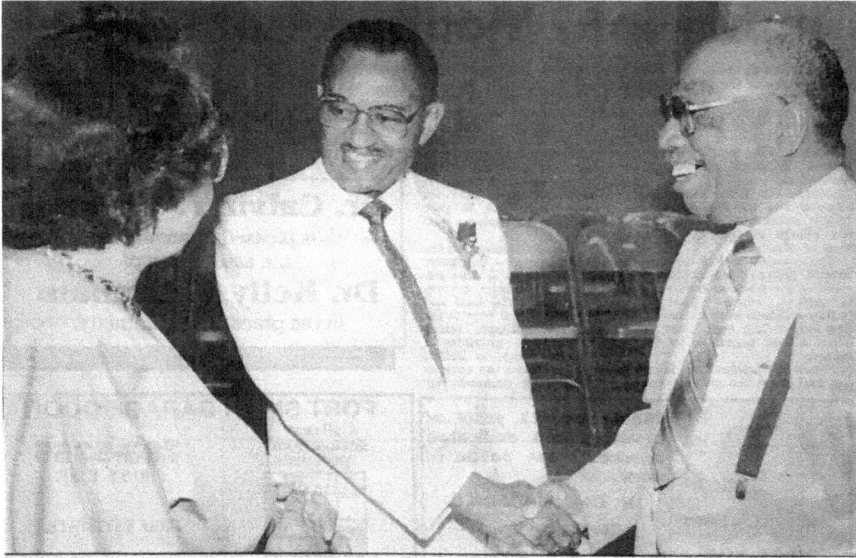

Harry in his white linen suit at his retirement party (Photo courtesy of Pebley Center, UAFS)

Harry said he had been doing some missionary work in Haiti, and he spent a month a year in Mexico. He was working on the genealogy of his family and had gone to Paris to track down the Deschamps family. His grandmother's father was a Deschamps, and he added that the Deschamps family had been surprisingly helpful, in view of the connection being from the offspring of their ancestor and one of his slaves. He had a cousin who also had some white ancestry, he said, and they weren't quite so helpful.

And so, I realized that Harry and I had a bit more in common than I had thought; he and I both grew up in the segregated rural South; we both moved to Fort Smith to practice medicine; and we were both descended from white southern slave owners.

"He knew who he was," Euba Winton told me. He certainly did, but I think that his interest in his family history was an extension of his lifelong concern to know more about who he was.

"He was a complicated person," Palmer recalls. "He loved life more than anybody I ever knew, and he loved people. But there was about twenty percent of him that was private. He didn't say everything he thought." The demands of practice didn't

139

leave much time for developing private interests—medicine, after all, is a jealous mistress—and in retirement he could take time for golf. "Maria likes to play golf, and he and Maria really bonded over golf," Palmer said. And then there were also art, music, and genealogy.

Harry's parents had good health into their mid-nineties, and Harry expected to do so, too. He was disciplined about his personal health. "His brother in Kansas City was a hard charger," Palmer continued. "He chain-smoked and drank coffee all the time, thirty cups a day. He worked twelve hours a day, had a busier practice and had more patients than Dad did. He had a bigger life, but Dad didn't envy him. He was happy being himself. But when Bruce got lung cancer in 1968, my dad stopped smoking and drinking—except for an occasional glass of wine with a meal. He said it was because his brother died."

Ill health came as a surprise to Harry, Palmer said, and his last years were melancholy ones as he dealt with multiple myeloma and cancer of the prostate. He had always had music in every room in the house, to keep his mood up—Earth Wind and Fire, Motown. He had everything on CD's. But from age eighty to eighty-eight he never listened to music.

Two events provided hope and affirmation during his health problems. Harry and Ruby had moved to Richland, Washington, to be near Maria, his youngest child. During the presidential campaign in 2008, Barrack Obama made a campaign stop an hour from Richland. Maria had missed Hillary Clinton's campaign stop, but she took her father and Ruby to Obama's appearance in an auditorium. Harry and Ruby were seated in the handicapped section, and they were the only black people there. When Obama spotted Harry, he came over and shook his hand. When Obama was elected, Harry thought that was a signal that the civil rights campaign had finally been victorious. [21]

Maria knew that her father wanted to talk to his old friend Bill Clinton before he died, and she contacted Charlotte Tidwell, who initiated the chain of contacts that resulted in a telephone conversation on March 28, 2012, three weeks before Harry died on April 15. Clinton said that he was still grateful for all the help Harry had given him. "I was just a nobody from nowhere with no money for nothing," he said, "and you enrolled me in the NAACP at Mallalieu Methodist Church in 1974. So, when I ran for president, I was able to say that I had been a member of the NAACP for eighteen years."

Harry's voice was weak as he responded to the former president. But in that telephone call he was once again in touch with the world. And it allowed him to go out on a positive note. In the words of Euba Winton, he always knew who he was. He was an agent of change and a force for good. He was on a mission. And his mission field was Fort Smith.

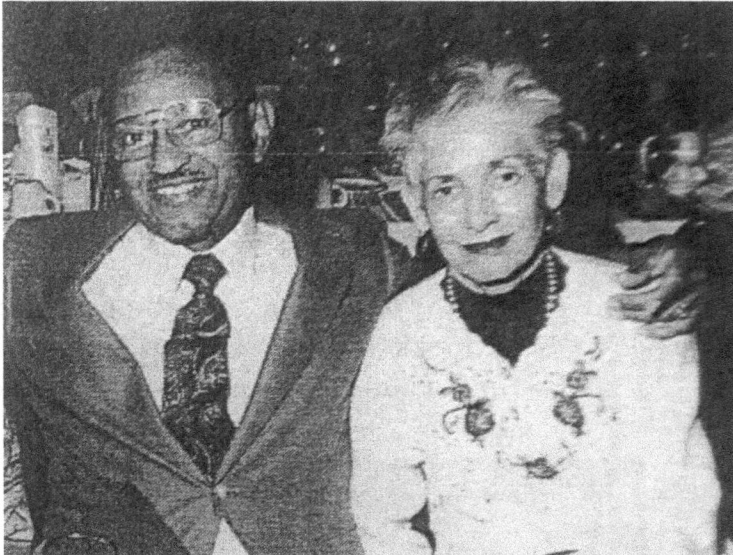

Harry & Ruby Bultman McDonald, his second wife (Photo courtesy of Pebley Center, UAFS

Ninety Percent Backbone

Roger Bost

After five years in practice in Fort Smith, Roger Bost told his partner John Watts that he wanted to run for the school board. Why? The superintendent would not allow children with disabilities to enroll. So: join the school board. As it turned out, he did win election to the school board, became its president two years later, and Fort Smith became the first school in the state to allow children with learning disabilities to enroll and participate in special education classrooms. Such an approach to challenges would in later years lead an opponent in the state legislature to say, "For such a runt of a man, he's ninety percent backbone."

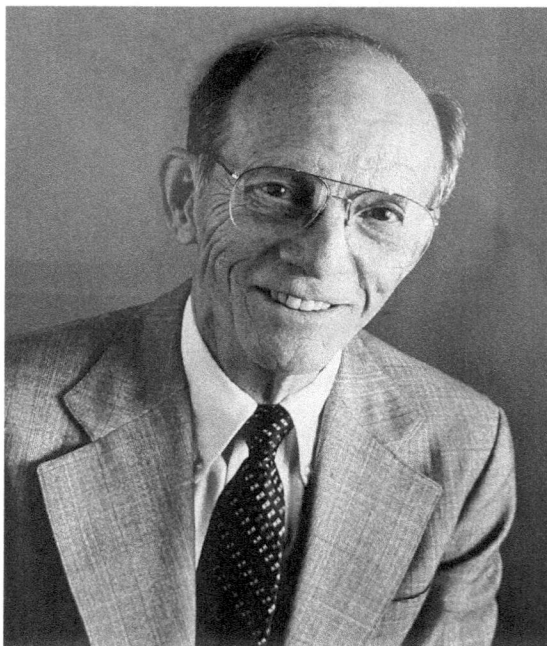

Roger B. Bost (BOST, Inc. Headquarters)

People in Fort Smith may also have said when he left town in 1965 to join the faculty at University of Arkansas Medical School, "His shoes aren't very big, but he sure does leave a big footprint." Not many physicians can put everything they have into taking care of patients and into public advocacy—not to mention family

142

responsibilities. The math doesn't add up. Roger Bost was one of those who made it add up. But it does require allocation of time and energy, and a willingness to change one's platform when necessary to be an effective agent of change.

Roger Browning Bost received his middle name from an ancestor, Captain John Browning, who made five voyages across the Atlantic to bring his family to Jamestown, Virginia, starting in 1620. A couple of centuries later, both his father's and mother's families came west from Hickory, North Carolina, to settle in Arkansas. [1] There weren't very many options in the Arkansas Territory, and one of them was around Clarksville in the Arkansas River Valley area, where, another century later, Roger was born October 28, 1921. His father, Roger Stone Bost, had graduated in the "first or second" [2] class of the University of Arkansas Pharmacy Department in 1912, opened a drugstore in Mulberry, and then moved twenty-five miles to the courthouse square in Clarksville nine years later.

"Everything I ever knew about pharmacy—and about life, really—began working in that old store," Dr. Bost recalled. "I remember jerking sodas there, running errands and all kinds of assorted tasks growing up. Then we'd close late at night and walk home." He attended the University of Arkansas and then transferred to College of the Ozarks in Clarksville where he could pay more attention to a childhood classmate, Kathryn King, whom he married in 1944 when he was a student at the University of Arkansas Medical School. (Kathryn graduated from College of the Ozarks in 1943.) After graduation from medical school in 1945 he served in the U.S. Navy, serving at Corpus Christi, Texas. After the war he was transferred to the Veterans Administration Hospital in Fayetteville.

Upon discharge from the Navy, he went to Duke University for a pediatric residency, then joined the Duke faculty in pediatrics. By 1951 he and Kathryn were beginning their family, and they moved to New Orleans, where he was associate professor of pediatrics at Tulane and was on the staff at Oschner Clinic and at Charity Hospital. It was in New Orleans that he developed a gastric ulcer and had a gastrectomy, which may have played a role in his maintaining a slender build for the rest of his ninety-two years.

After three years at Tulane, he elected to leave academia and go into private practice in Fort Smith, where he established the third pediatric practice in Arkansas. Dr. John Watts, who became Dr. Bost's partner in 1962, credits Dr. R.A. "Bud" Downs, a Fort Smith urologist at the time, with persuading Dr. Bost to come to Fort Smith. Dr. Pearl Waddell, a board-certified pediatrician who had practiced at Holt-Krock Clinic since 1932, was preparing to move to St. Simons Island,

Georgia, and when Dr. Watts arrived a few years later, he found himself so swamped with patients that it took him months to unpack his books. They made hospital rounds twice a day and many house calls. When the oral polio vaccine became available, they both drove house to house administering the vaccine.

Kathryn brought Roger his supper at the hospital if he was stuck there taking care of a sick child. He enjoyed driving a Karmann Ghia sports car, rationalizing that he spent more time in the car making house calls than anywhere else. His house calls as recalled by the children and parents were legendary, including the story that on one occasion he successfully retrieved a cat that had ventured too far out on the limb of a tree, and no one could get it down.

After beginning his practice on the second floor of a commercial building on Garrison Avenue, Dr. Bost retained Calvin Schriver, a local builder, to design and construct an office building on the corner of Fourth and D Streets, between Sparks and St. Edward hospitals. It has been described as having a "unique butterfly roof and Taliesin West-inspired structural members," creating "an eye-catching design that would stand out in any city . . . The use of large spans of clerestory windows around the building allowed for ample natural light in all of the exam rooms but also provided maximum privacy for the patients." [3]

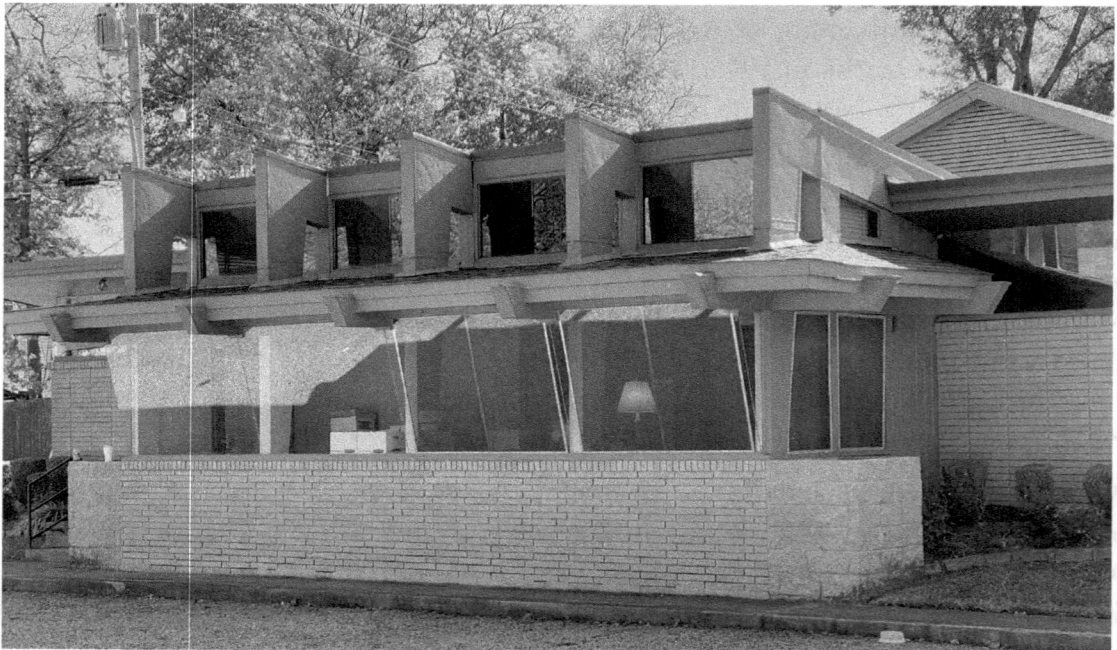

Bost Clinic in Fort Smith (Photo by author)

144

His office had a single waiting room for Blacks and whites. (He and Dr Davis Goldstein at Cooper Clinic were the two doctors known to have initiated this practice.) On one occasion he called one of the local hospitals to admit a Black child, knowing that the hospital's policy was not to admit Blacks. Upon being refused, he called one supervisor after another until he reached the chairman of the hospital board. He too refused. "You'll live to see the end of this hateful policy," Bost responded.

While maintaining such a busy practice, Roger enjoyed spending time talking to people, and as he listened, he became aware of community health issues that he wanted to address. One of his first projects was to provide support for children who were physically, mentally, or emotionally disabled. He personally solicited funds for a Child Family Guidance Center to treat emotional and behavioral problems and a day School for Limited Children for the developmentally disabled. "He went up and down the town, hat in hand, asking for donations from local shopkeepers to make it a reality," [4] recalled Kent Jones, a former director of BOST, Inc., a school that began in 1959 with six students in the basement of a house the First Methodist Church used for Sunday School classes. The Child Family Guidance Center became the Western Arkansas Counselling and Guidance Center, which has expanded to seven locations in western Arkansas, offering a variety of services including a special suicide prevention service.

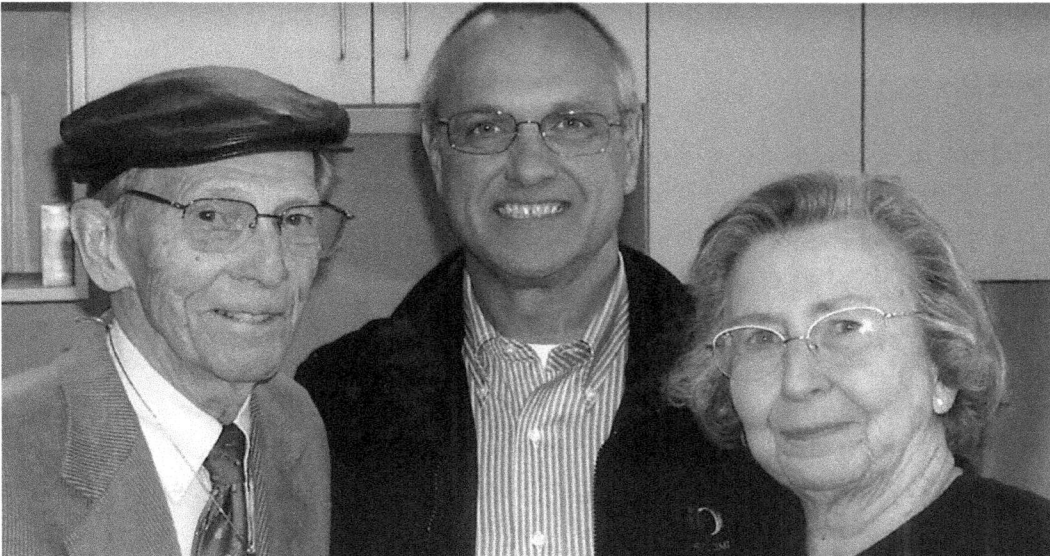

Kent Jones, Director of BOST with Roger and Katherine Bost (Photo from BOST Inc.)

145

The School for Limited Children became BOST, Inc. now with locations in twenty-eight counties in Arkansas, serving thousands of individuals of all ages. Katie Raines, current director of BOST, reports that its services include children's services with therapy, adult day treatment services teaching life skills and preparation for employment, and intermediate care in group settings. The largest program is home- and community-based, serving those who live at home but require anywhere from an hour to twenty-four hours a day support. A more recent service addresses mental health. [5]

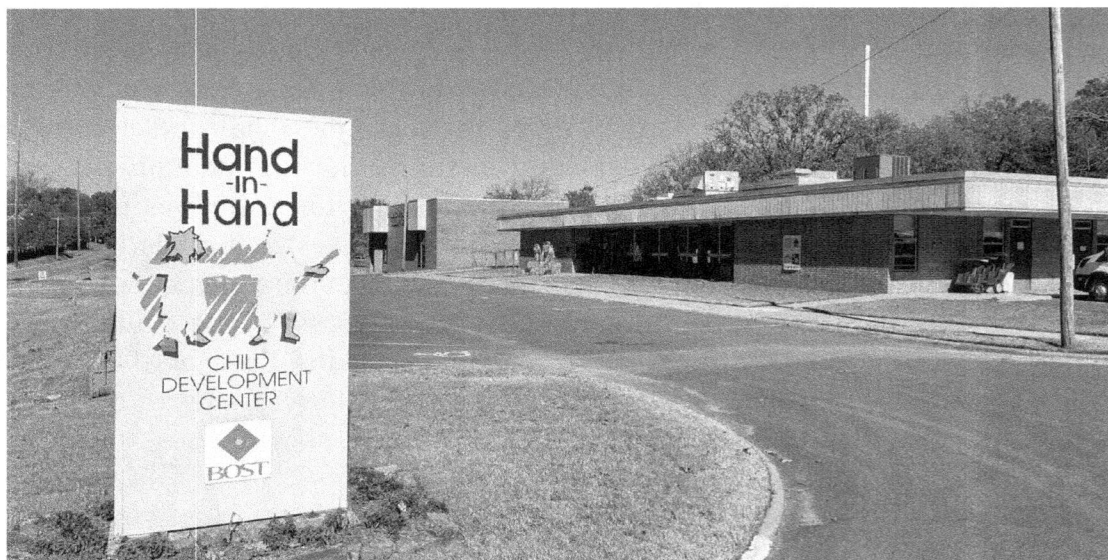

Child Development Center of BOST, Inc. in Fort Smith (Photo by author)

BOST, Inc. now owns two apartment complexes, three group homes and two intermediate care facilities. There is an apartment complex in Northwest Arkansas that is expanding because of the housing shortage there, and an intermediate care facility in Booneville.

At a fifty-year anniversary dinner in Fort Smith in 2009, Dr. Bost, though unable to attend, used a video to muse about the growth of BOST: "In 1959 from a tiny acorn (only six clients) a giant oak tree has grown (now serving seven hundred consumers in thirty-three counties)." He also remembered the financial support of the Junior Civic League over the years: "I think they emptied their treasury to get this program started," he said.

The Bosts had five children: Kingsley, now a pediatrician in Poplar Bluff, Missouri; Becky and Margaret, both now in Little Rock; Virginia, now in Russellville; and

Kevin Gao, now in New York City. Their home was on South 24th Street, and Virginia recalls Fort Smith at that time as a place where she could ride her bicycle anywhere she wanted to, with a wide open neighborhood that she could play in.

Amid all his community service, however, (for which his honors included the Book of Golden Deeds award), Dr. Bost's public role in health care in Arkansas had hardly begun. In 1965 the family moved to Little Rock where he resumed his academic career as an associate professor of pediatrics at UAMS. Continuing his interest in disabled children, he became administrator and medical director of the Crippled Children's Hospital in Little Rock. This was a time of flux in pediatric care, with the Arkansas Children's Hospital becoming the pediatrics department of UAMS and all pediatric patients at UAMS being moved to the Children's Hospital, which absorbed the patients of the Arkansas Crippled Children's Hospital as well.

When in practice in Fort Smith, Dr. Bost had taken care of the daughter of Dale and Betty Bumpers, nearby in Charleston. The young girl had a tumor of the spine, and Dr. Bost referred her to a colleague in neurosurgery whom he had known at Duke. She had successful surgery for her tumor at a New England medical center. Dr. Bost and Dale Bumpers became good friends, and after Bumpers was elected governor in 1970, he asked Bost to serve in his administration. They worked to create the Department of Social and Rehabilitation Services, today known as the Department of Human Services. This was a bruising legislative fight in which Bost's "ninety percent backbone" stood him in good stead.

Early on the agenda was a bill sponsored by Rep. Bill Stancil, who had been Fort Smith schools' first athletic director, to allow schools to accept disabled students. Bumpers also pushed through a bill driven by Bost and Arch Ford, Education Commissioner, requiring all Arkansas schools to educate disabled students, in regular classrooms when possible, and mandating the state to pay for it. [6]

"With Bost's tenacity and Bumpers' political magic," the legislature agreed to make use of federal Medicare and Medicaid funds which had been available but untapped, except for nursing home funds, since the creation of Medicare in 1965. "Medical services . . . were extended to the disabled and many others, including poor pregnant and nursing women; the state eventually quintupled the children's colonies and spread them around the state."

Having lived in Charleston, Bumpers was determined to make health care more widely available in rural areas. With Bost's help, UAMS increased its class size and awarded scholarships to students who would pledge themselves to practice for a time in a small town. Despite the opposition of the Arkansas Medical Society and the state medical board, they narrowly won approval for osteopaths to receive hospital and pharmacy privileges.

During his time of service in the Capitol, he saw the state Medicaid program grow from $10 million a year to $126 million a year; he oversaw the creation of community mental health centers throughout the state; and prescription drug coverage through Medicaid funds was introduced.

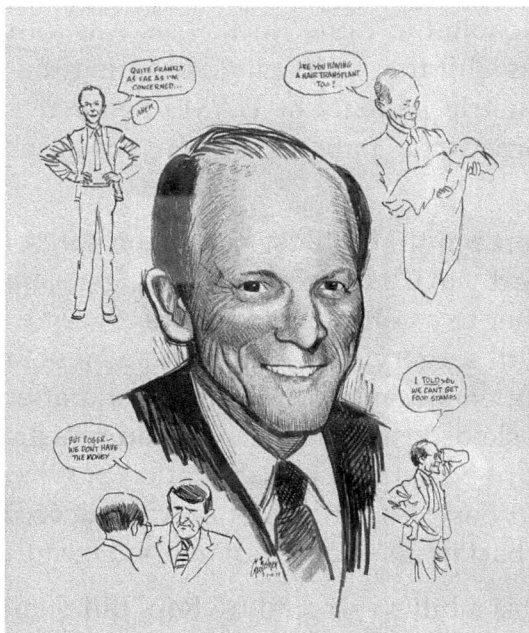

*Cartoon by George Fischer of the **Arkansas Gazette***

Bost returned to UAMS in 1975 as professor of pediatrics and associate dean of the college of medicine. In this capacity he designed the network of Area Health Education Centers (AHEC) in 1976 to expand fundamental health services in rural areas. One of the earliest of these was in Fort Smith. Others are in Batesville, Fayetteville, Helena, Jonesboro, Magnolia, Pine Bluff and Texarkana. This required a good bit of personal diplomacy in enlisting the support of local medical and community leaders. Such things don't just happen because someone in Little Rock signs a piece of paper.

His daughter Virginia Berner has told me about riding with her father to catch a plane. Seeing that the plane had already begun taxiing toward the runway as they drove up to the airport, they drove to the side of the runway where Bost got out, caught the pilot's eye and hailed him down. The plane stopped on the runway, and he boarded. Such was air travel in the good old days.

Bill Clinton became ill and called Dr. Bost, whom he only knew by reputation, on the night before his announcing his candidacy for governor in 1978, to ask for help. Despite Bost's protestations that he was a pediatrician, he did prescribe medication (probably children's aspirin), and Clinton made his announcement. Hillary Clinton attributed the improvement to "Bill's pediatrician."

When Dr. Harry Ward was named chancellor of UAMS to succeed Dr. William Shorey, Dr. Bost was the runner-up candidate. Though disappointed, Dr. Bost escorted Dr. Ward throughout the state introducing him to his own contacts, and Bost and Ward became fast friends. Bost then, at age seventy-two, returned to the practice of pediatrics at Arkansas Children's Hospital, where he developed the Children's Care Center, modeling it after his own clinic he had built in Fort Smith. He retired from this position, and though he returned for short post-retirement stints, he began to decline these opportunities to spend more time on the golf course. Other interests included dogs, pocketknives, hats, picking fruit, the Arkansas Razorbacks, and the St. Louis Cardinals, and he never went anywhere without an apple and peanut butter crackers. He was a Methodist and a Democrat.

I met him one time, when we both happened to be at a funeral in Little Rock in 2010. These are my notes from the meeting:

> A lady standing nearby introduced herself as Kathryn Bost; her husband Roger was around and came over later. He was very gracious. "Oh, yes, I know you, Taylor. I've kept up with you. You were a breath of fresh air when you came to Fort Smith."
> He told us he practiced in Fort Smith from 1955 to 1965 before going to Little Rock where he was head of pediatrics at Arkansas Children's Hospital. And later Dale Bumpers and David Pryor had him be head of the state health department. He's eighty-nine now—says he doesn't know why he's still around—he's rather small, partially bald, wore a semi-turtleneck shirt and tweed jacket. A few stories from his Fort Smith days: John Watts joined him in his practice, and when John called, during his search, Roger asked Kathryn what John's wife's name was. She didn't remember—some sort of precious stone—so he asked John, "How's Opal?" I think Garnet has told us that story.
> When he first came, Prentiss and Gladys Ware invited them to a party they were having, and Gladys took him around introducing him to the others. When she got to McLeod Sicard (president of the First National Bank), McLeod said, "Pediatrics? Well, you'll sure be busy. Everybody's got foot problems."

Roger Bost was a charter member of the UAMS Hall of Fame in 2004. He died November 19, 2013, at age ninety-two, at his home in Little Rock. After his funeral at St. James United Methodist Church in Little Rock, he was buried in Clarksville, his birthplace.

Ernest Dumas characterized Dr. Bost in his obituary notice in *The Arkansas Times*:

> A less imposing man would be hard to find. Frail, short, bespectacled and bald at an early age, Roger Bost's mortal frame was outfitted with a voice so thin and reedy that he could barely be heard above the muted whispers in the legislative hearing rooms where he often spoke forty years ago.
>
> But, boy, did he get heard. No one in Arkansas ever did as much to lift the welfare of children, and not just children but people of all ages who at some point have found themselves or loved ones outside the latitudes of first-rate health care or social services. That may include most of Arkansas. [7]

Just Before It Got Complicated

A Personal Memoir of the Early 1970s

The Lay of the Land

"Taylor, last Sunday morning at seven o'clock I saw you running from Sparks to St. Edward on Lexington Avenue. There wasn't much light, but you had your white coat on, and your coattails were flying." One of my colleagues (who must have also been on call that weekend) told me this, and I can't deny it. My recollection is vague, and I have no idea about the details—like why I wasn't driving my car. Yet I was spotted by a credible witness. I do know that I was fit enough and young enough and crazy enough to be doing such a thing. But one point of this shadowy recollection is that the old St. Edward on Fifteenth and Rogers, and the "old" Sparks, in its 1970 iteration and before it was completely turned around and at least doubled in size, were not that far apart, geographically or in any of the many other ways they drifted apart in subsequent years.

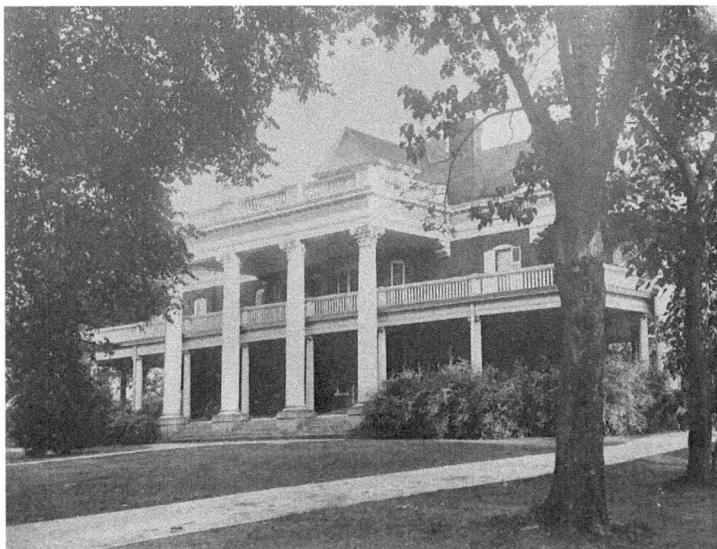

This building on 1500 Dodson was built in 1890 by Dr. J. H. T. Main, one of the first physicians in Fort Smith, for his daughter and her husband Dr. Worth Bailey. It became the Colonial Hospital in 1929 when it changed hands, and when the Colonial Hospital closed in 1952 it was purchased by Holt-Krock Clinic. The house was demolished and replaced by a new clinic building in 1977—which is now Baptist Health Plaza. (Photo from Reference 11 – Present at the Creation)

Holt-Krock Clinic was only a couple of blocks from Sparks, and Cooper Clinic only a block from St. Edward; and this geographical connection was supported by various informal and unspoken considerations. Charles Holt, founder of Holt-Krock Clinic, was the owner of the old St. John's Hospital when he closed it in 1934 and merged it with Sparks, where he served as the administrator of the hospital. One of his daughters became the wife of Marvin Altman, a later administrator of Sparks (starting as business manager in 1939 and retiring as president in 1979). Holt-Krock physicians routinely held staff leadership positions at Sparks. Lou Lambiotte was head of the internal medicine department at Sparks when I came in 1969 and continued in that role for many years.

Even less structured was the relationship between St. Edward and Cooper Clinic. For one thing, St. Edward was of course Catholic, and Cooper Clinic, with two of its founders being Jewish, was decidedly secular. Everett Foster, one of the founders of Cooper Clinic, was the first chief of staff at St. Edward, a position often filled by other Cooper Clinic physicians. People in town often assumed the association between hospitals and clinics to be closer than it was, and whenever people asked me about my affiliations, it often required a sentence or two to explain that I worked at Cooper Clinic and not for St. Edward.

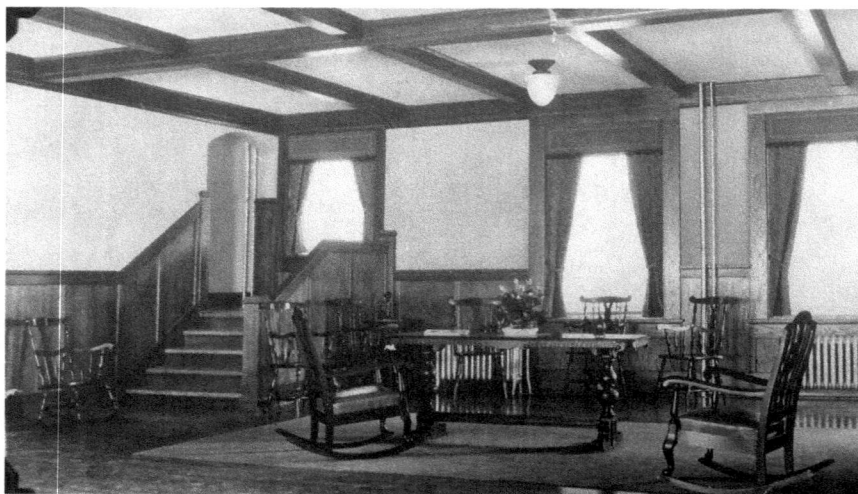

Built in 1924 the Cooper Clinic building on 1400 South 11th featured rocking chairs in its lobby. Cooper Clinic moved out of the building in 1972, and it was later demolished. (Photo hangs in Mercy Tower West)

Whenever one of my patients needed to be hospitalized, in my early years of practice, I routinely asked them their choice, and the split was about sixty percent St. Edward and forty percent Sparks. I referred patients to my Cooper Clinic partners as a matter of policy (after being gently reminded about this by one of my senior partners after one or two early transgressions), but otherwise my policy was to refer to the "best in town," as another of my senior partners described his policy when it was necessary to send a patient outside the clinic.

I became good friends with independent and Holt-Krock physicians as we made rounds at St. Edward and Sparks. A certain bit of rivalry was inevitable, but as in so many other things, "you had to cooperate to graduate," and collegiality trumped competition.

The Old Hospitals

The old St. Edward, now the Mid-Town Apartments, was distinctive in several ways. To begin with, there were the nuns, who ran the place. Most were senior, and they were authoritative. Sister Judith Marie Keith was still a young woman when she became the administrator in 1970; she was energetic, cheerful, and competent, but so were her senior sisters. For instance, Sister Albertine oversaw the operating room, and her authority was such that on at least one occasion when she postponed a surgical case because she did not consider the surgeon to be at his best that day, nobody questioned her, including the surgeon himself.

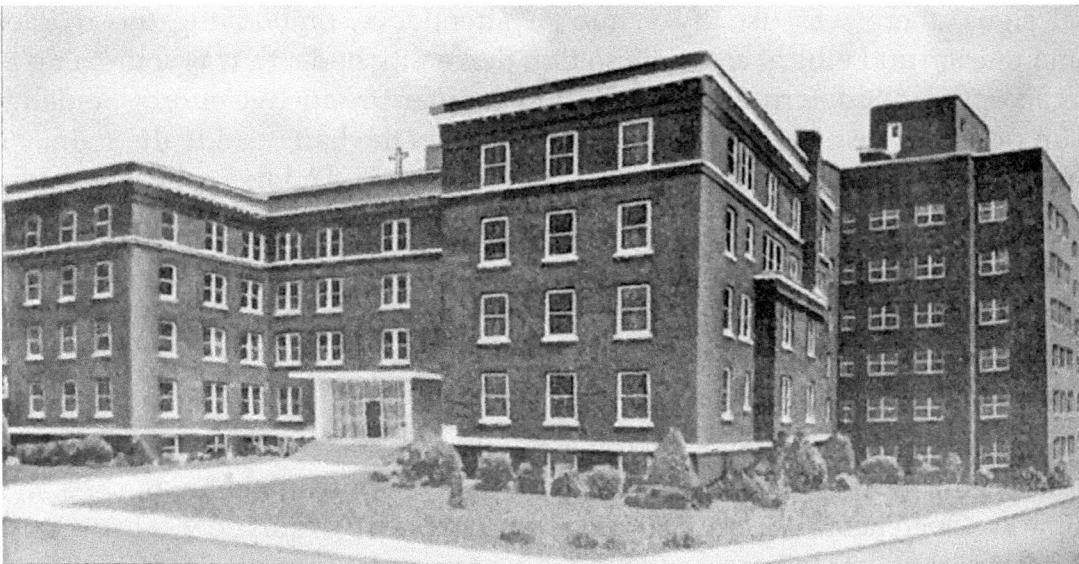

This postcard photo shows the St. Edward hospital that was built in 1922. An annex, shown on the right, was added in 1953. Since St. Edward moved to South 74th Street in 1975, the building has been occupied by Midtown Apartments.

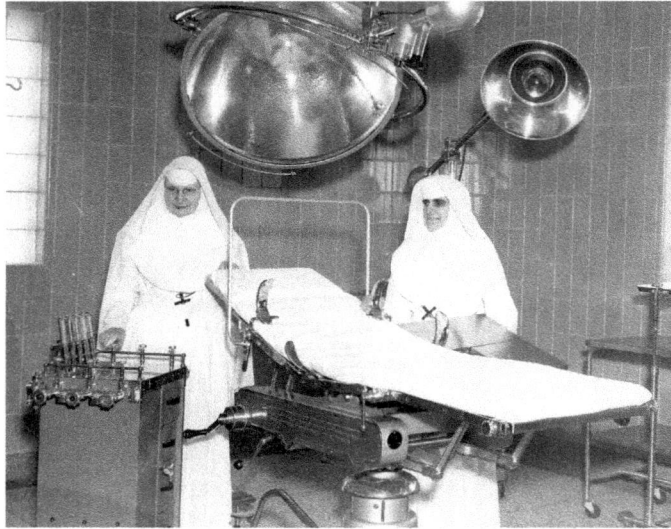

Sister Sebastian, on the left, and Sister Albertine on the right, are shown in the fifth-floor operating room of St Edward when it was on 15th and Rogers. (Photo from Mercy archives).

With the nuns in attendance, the mode of dying was different. There were no living wills, no ethics committees, very few code blues (although we were beginning to introduce cardiopulmonary resuscitation [CPR] in the intensive care unit, sometimes with surprising success). When a dying patient ceased to have vital signs, there was usually a nun in attendance, embodying the religious, humanitarian and ethical concerns so that the reality of death was something that was accepted, not deferred with futile and counter-productive efforts. Sometimes a nun or a priest would quietly murmur to me in the hall outside the room, "It's time for him (or her) to go to heaven, isn't it, Doctor?" And the issue was settled.

I found that as a young Methodist doctor some of the authority of the Church rubbed off on me. As I was explaining her condition to a faithful Catholic woman, she responded, "Yes, Doctor." "Yes, Doctor." "Yes, Doctor." "Yes, Father—I mean Yes, Doctor." Alas, such unquestioning acceptance of the authority of the doctor didn't last much longer than the doctors' universal wearing of suits.

The old Sparks may not have had nuns, but it had its own features. When I joined Cooper Clinic in 1969, interventional cardiology was already being pushed ahead at Sparks. Open heart surgery had been begun by a trio of surgeons—Leon Woods of Holt-Krock; Carl Williams, an independent practitioner; and Eddie Clemmons, who was in Cooper Clinic at that time. They started in the animal lab before offering the procedure to local patients, with the doctor sitting up all night in the patient's room in intensive care on at least the first night after surgery.

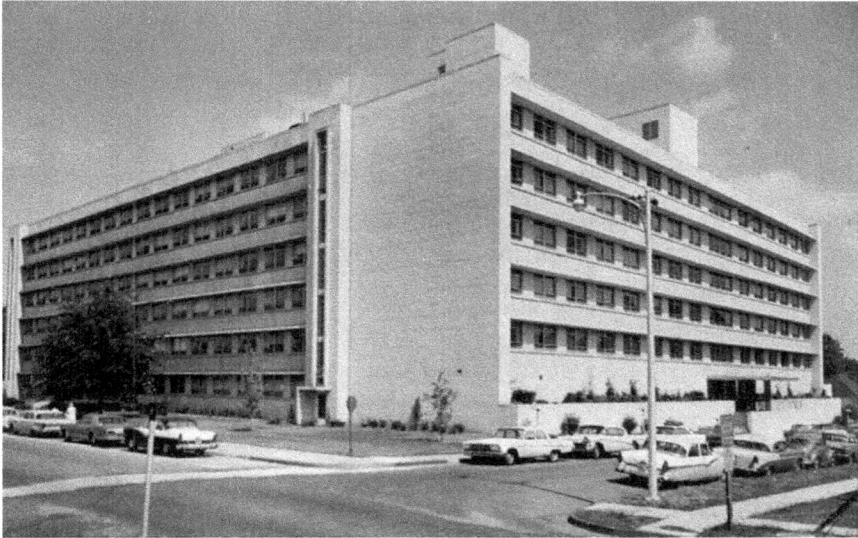

This postcard photograph shows Sparks as it stood in 1953 when this 150-bed facility was opened. Another wing was added in 1966, and when a new 206-bed East Wing was added in 1979, Sparks became for a time the largest hospital in Arkansas.

Cardiac catheterization was a prerequisite for coronary artery bypass and for valvular surgery, and Keith Klopfenstein had begun the cath lab at Sparks. He joined Holt-Krock in 1963, the first cardiologist in Fort Smith.

Radiology was another part of the cardiac surgery project, and the radiologists at Sparks forged ahead with interpretation of coronary arteriograms. Weekly cardiac conferences were held at Sparks, at which surgeons, cardiologists from both clinics, and radiologists reviewed coronary arteriograms and other data on candidates for surgery and determined management plans.

Another unique attraction at Sparks was the dining room; doctors and their families routinely ate Sunday dinner at Sparks after church. Charles Shuffield, CEO of Sparks from 1979 to 1997, told me that his predecessor, Marvin Altman, told him that if he fed the doctors well, he would get along fine. Current staff members assure me that even though the hospital has had several changes of ownership, the Altman Doctrine is still well observed.

Hospital Rounds

Intensive care units began to appear in medical centers in the 1960s; the first ones were specialized—a trauma and burn unit, a postoperative neurosurgical unit.

155

When I arrived in Fort Smith in 1969, Sparks and St. Edward each had a general intensive care unit. These early ICUs evolved on an ad hoc basis; Sparks had an early need for specialized care for patients who had had open heart surgery, so there was one section designated as the cardiac ICU, which also provided care for patients with myocardial infarctions (heart attacks).

Intensive care was intense, but otherwise hospital care was more leisurely in the seventies. Nobody worried about length of stay. As an isolated and extreme example, for years we shared among ourselves the story of one of us getting a call on a Thursday or Friday, from a nurse at Sparks. "Doctor, we have a patient on our floor who was admitted by one of your partners on Sunday. He's doing okay, but I don't think a doctor's been in to see him yet." It turned out that a doctor on call had admitted a patient on a Sunday, taken off on vacation the next day, and left this patient's name off the list he turned in to his partners. The head nurse kept an eye on the patient, reassured him that all was well, and that the doctor would be in soon. After three or four days, she decided it was time to make a phone call.

The head nurses ran their floors in authoritarian fashion, some colorfully so. When one of my younger partners was making his first visit to a certain floor at Sparks, the head nurse saw that he was new and took him aside. "Sonny boy," she said, and then she paused. "You do just what I tell you and you'll be all right."

"Yes, ma'am."

Doctors also wielded unchecked power in some ways. It was a shock to come to Fort Smith in 1969 and discover that I could admit any patient I wanted to, for any reason, at any time. In training I had to funnel each admission past an admitting resident, whose vested interest was to allow no admissions at all. But here, the nurses said, "Yes, sir," and that was it. People were often admitted for diagnostic examinations that are now done on an outpatient basis because insurance companies and hospitals have discovered that it's cheaper that way. This was in the days before gastroscopy and colonoscopy, and patients were often admitted for an upper GI series and a barium enema, x-ray procedures that required administration of a barium liquid material. A patient may not have been feeling well or may have needed a rest—whatever. And the concept of "length of stay" had not yet been invented. Stay as long as you like. We're happy to have you.

Patients were admitted to the hospital at least one day before surgery for studies that are now done routinely on an outpatient basis. Among other things, a primary care doctor was asked to see the patient in the hospital the night before surgery for "pre-op clearance." This could be a big part of the evening for an internist connected with a busy surgical group; there might be half a dozen or more of these on a busy night. One internist who left Fort Smith for a group practice elsewhere told me later, with some satisfaction, that his new group had three surgeons and eighteen internists—with emphasis on the "eighteen," meaning that his evenings were no longer dominated by a chore that had become increasingly burdensome for him.

In talking to the family after a death, we were trained to ask the family for permission to have an autopsy done. I would explain that it would help us to know for sure what the cause of death was; and although it couldn't change anything in this case, it would help us in the care of others in the future. This was a difficult question to ask, and it was easier to just let it go; and as diagnostic techniques improved so that we had CT scans and MRIs and other tests that made us think we knew more about what was going on, autopsies became less frequent and are now rarely done. But in the 1970s doctors knew where the morgue was, because we went down there (in every hospital, it always seemed to be in an obscure corner of the basement) when an autopsy was being done, and the pathologist would show us his findings; and the doctor would report to the family.

Appearances were different in the 1970s. Doctors wore white coats in their offices but wore suits and ties when making rounds in the hospitals. Smoking was prevalent among doctors, nurses, and patients in the hospitals. Cigarettes were left burning on a stand in the hall when the doctor entered a patient's room (usually). Nurses wore caps, and they did not wear pants. Scrubs were limited to the operating room. Nursing students in their special blue uniforms were seen on the nursing floors. St. Edward had at least four four-bed wards.

One doctor who never gave up his cigars was Dr. W.R. (Bill) Brooksher, director of the department of radiology at St. Edward. (He started practice in Fort Smith with his father, who specialized in surgery and radiology, and he served as editor of the *Journal of the Arkansas Medical Society* from 1933 to 1944.) Dr. Brooksher was in the hospital's x-ray room with a cigar in his hand when one of the surgeons came in with an "IQ" lapel button.

"What does that 'IQ' mean?"

"I Quit. I've quit smoking. I've saved a lot of money."

"You must have. Got it all in the bank, I suppose?"

Not all the doctors were white males. Sarah Jennings, an internist at Holt-Krock, was one of the six new doctors who arrived in Fort Smith in 1969. Annette

Landrum had her own pathology practice, and I regularly saw Dr. Louise Henry, who practiced ophthalmology with her husband Dr. Murphy Henry, at Sparks staff meetings. I don't remember any other women in practice in Fort Smith at that time. The only African American physician was Dr. Harry McDonald (see "He Knew Who He Was").

A Little Help from One's Friends

There were fewer doctors at that time; we all had more than enough to do, and there was a sense of community. We saw one another making rounds at both hospitals, and there was a good bit of shop talk. Friendships were not limited to one's partners.

In late 1969 three of us who were young internists decided to form a "journal club." Bill Turner, hematologist at Holt-Krock, had retained his academic enthusiasm after having trained at Johns Hopkins, and he was delighted to meet with me and Larry Price, who had been my classmate and neighbor at Washington University in St. Louis. Larry and I had gone in different directions for training and military duty—Larry spent a year in Vietnam—and when we began looking for practice locations, we discovered that we were both headed to Fort Smith. Larry joined Zach Hornberger and Hugh Lewing in a partnership. He and I both started to work in the same city on the same day, July 1, 1969, and we continued to be colleagues and the best of friends in different practice arrangements. Our journal club met monthly at one home or another, and we tried to keep our conversation centered on the articles each of us was presenting, but of course a little shop talk slipped in.

Jerry Stewart joined Cooper Clinic in July 1970, and he became a fourth member of our journal club. During the ten years or so of its existence, our meetings sometimes swelled to ten or twelve, with colleagues from independent practices and both clinics.

Professional roles and responsibilities were a bit blurred at a time when some lines had not yet been defined. I was a cardiologist, but I shared call and patients with two general internists. Having been recently certified in general internal medicine as a prerequisite to cardiology certification, I was happy to see and do anything other internal medicine doctors did. I did not become involved in surgery, although my partner, Jerry Stewart, did have at least one such opportunity when he was called in the middle of the night by Wright Hawkins, senior surgeon at Cooper Clinic. Dr. Hawkins needed him to assist in surgery at Sparks, and so the pulmonary medicine specialist, who was not even on call for internal medicine that night, held a retractor for a general surgeon at three o'clock in the morning.

These were the days before emergency room doctors, and the emergency room at night, particularly the eleven-to-seven shift, was the unquestioned domain of the head nurse, who made a triage judgment on every patient who came in, and when necessary, she called the doctor on call. One night I was called in at two a.m. to see a patient with abdominal pain, and as I was scratching my head as to whether it might be appendicitis, I decided to call Buddy Holmes, a general surgeon, just to ask his advice for what I needed to do to take care of the situation until morning. He gave me some suggestions, and I set to work. About twenty or thirty minutes later I looked up and Buddy was walking in the door. "I lay back down after I hung up the phone, and I just got curiouser and curiouser."

Office Calls

Even those of us who worked in the old Cooper Clinic at 100 South 14th Street can hardly believe that the building was squeezed into the tiny oblong lot adjoining the City National Bank, now Cadence Bank. From 1925 until 1972 the two-story red brick building (with a basement) housed a clinic with up to at least nine or ten physicians with waiting room, x-ray and lab, and business office; and there was still parking space behind the building for six doctors' cars. I worked there as a rookie physician from 1969 to 1972, when we moved into a new building way out on Waldron and Ellsworth, across from the new Central Mall— "out there with the wildcats," as one of our skeptical doctors said.

The downtown building represented medicine as I had encountered it as a boy, with oak or mahogany furnishings, a well-worn staircase, and nurses in crisp white uniforms and caps. This was a time when an office call was three dollars, a longer visit was five dollars, and a new patient examination was fifteen dollars. House calls were still an established custom; our charge was fifteen dollars, and on at least one occasion when I found myself visiting a traveler in a motel room, I collected in cash. X-rays and electrocardiograms were done just down the hall from the doctor's office, and the doctor looked at both with you before you left.

The Cooper Clinic building was the state of the art when it opened in 1924 to house a three-year-old multi-specialty clinic modelled after the still relatively new Mayo Clinic in Rochester, Minnesota. For a young doctor in a later generation, the last years of the red brick building on South 14th Street were an exciting time as the medical community was expanding with new talent coming into town in both

159

Cooper Clinic and the larger Holt-Krock Clinic at 1500 Dodson, and also in the independent medical sector. The building housed a lot of history, much of which I knew little of, but even the seemingly elastic walls that had stretched to accommodate three new doctors in 1969–70 would not be able to handle the three new doctors who would come in 1973, with more and more to follow.

Many in Fort Smith remember going to the original Cooper Clinic as children to see Drs. Miles Foster, Davis Goldstein, Sidney Wolferman, or some of the newer doctors, known for years as their "assistants": Drs. Ken Thompson, Wright Hawkins, and Calvin Bradford. Dr. Goldstein was the only one of the founders still living in 1969 when I came, and by then he had retired. My mentors were in the second generation, and some of Dr. Thompson's patients considered me his "assistant."

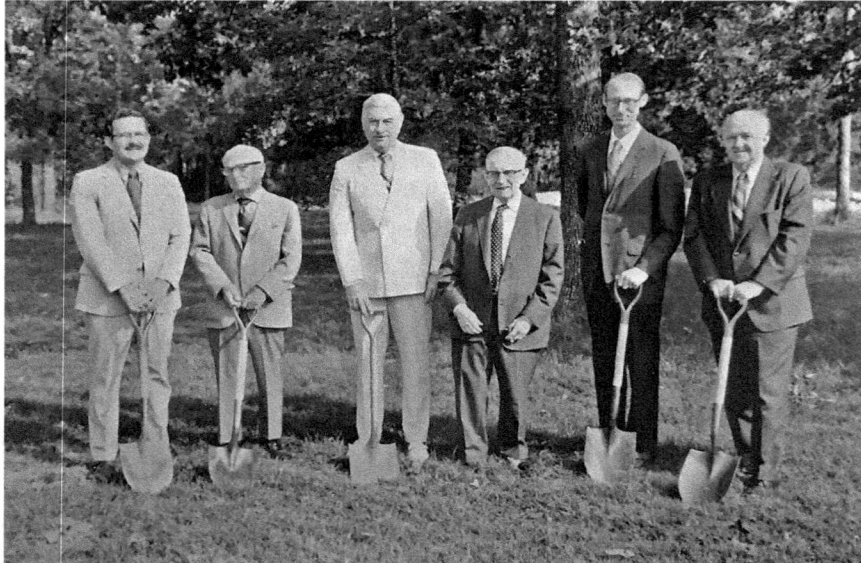

Cooper Clinic broke ground for its new clinic building on Waldron Road in 1971. Left to right: Dr. J.V. LeBlanc, Dr. Davis Goldstein, Dr. Ken Thompson, Dr. W.R. Brooksher, Dr. Taylor Prewitt, J.L. McAleb, clinic manager. (Photo from Cooper Clinic archives in Pebley Center, UAFS)

Dr. Thompson's appearance was distinguished; he was tall and well built, and with his silver hair and mustache, he could have played a Clifton Webb-like role in Hollywood as the prototype of the senior physician of the 1930s or 1940s. He would never have said so, but respect for the patient was one of his cardinal principles, and I learned this as much from his patients as from him. This was the time when a "physical" really was a physical examination. I may have thought that some of this was unnecessary ritual, but it became apparent to me that if the patient was paying the bill, I was obliged to give them their money's worth. As I was finishing an examination of one of Dr. Thompson's older patients, in his absence, she asked me, "Aren't you going to look in my eyes?" I didn't think that using the ophthalmoscope to peer into the patient's eyes was necessary on every examination, but this lady told me, "Dr. Thompson always looks in my eyes." So, of course, I did. She then asked me if something was wrong. No, I said, everything was just fine. "When Dr. Thompson looks in my eyes, he always tells me everything is fine." So that little word became part of my routine.

Doctors' schedules were a bit different from those of today. Internists at Cooper Clinic would make hospital rounds from about eight a.m. to nine thirty a.m., then see patients at the clinic. No patients were scheduled from noon to two p.m., and although morning patients routinely spilled over well past noon, we usually had time to go somewhere—maybe even home—for lunch. We then had clinic patients scheduled until five p.m. and made evening rounds.

A major change in delivery of health care occurred when Medicare became a fact of life in 1966, three years before I began practice, so I had no experience with life before Medicare. Health insurance, however, was not so prevalent and dominant as it is today, and I felt very keenly that people were paying real money for what I did, and it was my job to be sure they felt like they were getting good value for their money. Joe LeBlanc, my mentor in the facts of life, told me his response when a patient complained about his bill. "How much do you think it should be?" And whatever the answer, "Okay, that's what it is." Such was the sheltered life I led, however, that although I was prepared to use that answer, I don't think I ever had an opportunity.

Joe also explained his policy about seeing clergy and nuns. "I never charge a nun. I never charge a priest." Joe later moved away, and I inherited a number of his patients. A later partner, Bill Holman, said, "Taylor and I have an agreement. He sees all the preachers. I see all the drunks. I think I got the better end of the bargain." A good line, but some of my greatest blessings came from the lives of those who had chosen a life of service.

Answering the Calls

Returning telephone calls could sometimes be a chore, but Ken Thompson helped put it in perspective for those of us who complained about it. There was one woman who called him almost daily. It was not that he was her only physician.

"Sometimes she calls to ask me what another doctor meant by what he said when she saw him yesterday." Ken went home at noon, and after lunch he lay on his bed with a Princess telephone, a lightweight little receiver he had bought for the purpose, on his chest, returning his calls.

Ken's senior status qualified him to be a guardian of the traditional ways of doing things, and one of the first things I learned in private practice was that I should always drop whatever I was doing to answer a call from another doctor. This practice began to drift a bit before Ken retired, and one time he called one of the younger doctors during clinic hours and was told by the receptionist that the doctor would return his call later because he was in a room with a patient. Wrong answer. A thundering response. "Well, that's where he's supposed to be! Now get him on the phone!"

People often need medical attention after hours, and in some ways this process is unchanged after fifty years. The patient calls the office number, the answering service answers, they notify the doctor on call, and the patient receives a call from a doctor (or perhaps, nowadays, from a nurse practitioner). The process was a bit more primitive, and more personal, in the 1970s. The Cooper Clinic answering service was operated by a tireless woman who received patient calls and transmitted them to the doctor. This was before the era of personal pagers or cell phones, and she would call me at home, or at the hospital, or wherever else I might be. I let her know where I was when I was on call, and she would call me there. When making weekend hospital rounds, I would call every half hour or so to see if she was holding any calls for me, and then I would return the calls. Many of them involved a need for a prescription, and I knew the phone numbers of half a dozen or so pharmacies by heart. With a little effort, I can still almost remember the numbers for Prince Drug Store, Economy Drug, Coleman's Pharmacy, Laws Drug Store, Vaughn Prescription Drug, and other regulars. The pharmacists knew my voice, and I knew theirs, and there were no intermediary machines or numbers to dial. I regularly had symphony and other show seats on the aisle so I could scoot out more easily.

I learned to consider it a privilege to make house calls, but they could also be an inconvenient chore at times. Ken told about being summoned to see one of his neighbors who lived in a red brick mansion on Adelaide Street. He arrived rather promptly after being called in the middle of the day, to find two of our colleagues, Zach Hornberger and Kemal Kutait, also there. His neighbor had wanted to see someone in a hurry, so she called all three.

The clinic supplied me with a doctor's bag for making house calls. It was brown and shaped like a briefcase rather than the traditional black satchel. The clinic manager explained to me that if it looked less like a regular doctor's bag, it would be less likely to be stolen for drugs. It was indeed supplied with drugs—a vial or two of Demerol, but mostly with other necessities: Vistaril, a common and rather mild sedative for intramuscular injections; and a few other now outdated items for emergencies. The only one I remember using, however, was Vistaril. One woman often called on evenings when I was on call, saying her nerves were horrible and she needed a shot. After dutifully going to her house and administering an intramuscular injection once or twice, I complained to her regular doctor, that these trips and the shots were unnecessary at best. He listened patiently to my complaints, and his terse response anticipated the Nike slogan: "Just do it."

More often, however, the house call was worthwhile for the patient and rewarding to me as the doctor. I learned to know the patient and the family far better from seeing them in the home than from office or emergency room visits. It was often easier to move the doctor to the patient than to move the patient to the doctor. And on rare occasions the doctor would even move the patient to the hospital— carrying him to the car in the middle of the night on one occasion and driving him in. On another occasion I used the four-wheel drive option to fetch a woman with pericardial tamponade (a medical emergency) when the roads were icy.

In later years, and for as long as I was in practice, I sometimes volunteered to make a house call. This would surprise the patient; nobody thought that house calls were still being done. But it was sometimes easier for me to drop by on my way home after hospital rounds. And on one memorable occasion I made a quick drive to Ozark, some forty miles away, to see a patient in the hospital. The doctor had her reasons for keeping the patient in Ozark instead of transferring him, and I enjoyed a mid-day break from the local routine.

High Standards

From my colleagues I learned lessons big and small that I had not learned in medical school. My partners caught me up on various skills and techniques. Jerry Stewart, for example, taught me joint aspiration, and Tim Waack, in later years, taught me to do transesophageal echocardiography. And whenever I called Leon Woods for help, his voice would make me think that he had been waiting all day for me to call. No more names. There were too many, and I would leave out some that I should have mentioned.

I did learn, though, that as I tried to follow the example of Leon Woods and be friendly on the telephone, I had the opportunity to have more and more respect for the doctors in such towns as Charleston, Greenwood, Alma, Mulberry, Lavaca, Booneville, Paris, Clarksville, Ozark, Mena, Waldron—and also Oklahoma towns such as Sallisaw, Heavener, Poteau, Wilburton, Bokoshe, Stigler, and Vian. One learns a lot about doctors from their patients. The doctors in these areas were hard-working and dedicated, and I began to realize that they successfully took care of some pretty sick people; they knew when to hold 'em and knew when to fold 'em. Joe LeBlanc told me one evening just before my first day at the clinic, "Someday you will be bone tired after being up all night and all day; you'll finally finish seeing your last patient and be ready to go home and go to bed; and that's when Joe Roberts will call from Charleston and say he's sending you a patient in diabetic coma, with congestive heart failure and renal shutdown."

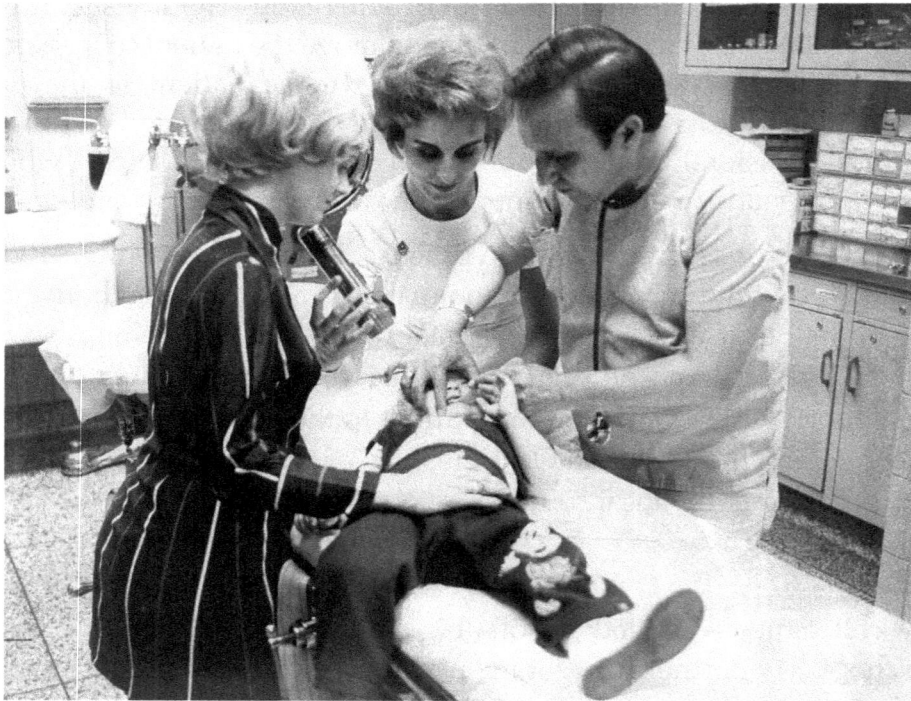

Agnes Locknar, night nurse in the 1970s St. Edward emergency room, decided when to call the doctor in.

I'm not sure I ever got that call. Joe Roberts became a good friend; he was one of those who practiced alone, took all his own calls, and took good care of his patients. Yes, I got pretty tired at times, but I wasn't the only one.

The quality of medical care in the 1970s, before President Ford came to Fort Smith and a doctor could whiz over from one hospital to the other on foot, was indeed very good. Having done my job-hunting in other good locations in the state, Fort Smith was the one that had the culture of a crossroads community, drawing physicians from Oklahoma and points west, Kansas City and points north, New Orleans and other points south, and Memphis and other points east. I had come a long way from St. Louis.

For a young doctor who wanted to take care of sick folks, it was Camelot.

Before closing this description of an otherwise somewhat idyllic system of delivery of health care, however, one issue has not been addressed: "Who took care of the poor folks?" Having seen a preponderance of the medically indigent in my years of schooling and training in St. Louis, Chapel Hill, and Memphis, I asked our clinic administrator this question. "There aren't any," he said. "We take care of everybody." This was wrong.

Oh, my colleagues and I took care of some who paid little or nothing. But this was a drop in the bucket. One scene comes to mind: I was called to a small frame house a block or two off Midland—not an upscale address—to see a seventeen-year-old African-American man who had fever and joint pains. There was also a heart murmur. This was acute rheumatic fever, a common disease of half a century earlier before penicillin and improved public health measures coincided with its almost complete disappearance. The house was hot, and there must have been six or eight family members crowded into the sickroom—a perfect culture medium for propagating a streptococcal infection. This brief description raises more issues than can be addressed here, but even though acute rheumatic fever may now be considered a third world disease, there are a host of other measures of health in which our nation lags notoriously behind other developed nations. I see examples of this every time I go to the Good Samaritan Clinic, a nonprofit entity providing health care access regardless of ability to pay. But volunteer agencies are a stopgap measure in the absence of a more comprehensive solution.

Epilogue

Though it did not seem so at the time, things moved quickly after 1975. Both hospitals grew, contracted, and changed their names. Sparks changed its ownership several times. Both clinics grew to over a hundred physicians, contracted, and disappeared. Doctors came, and doctors left. It begins to sound like the Grand Hotel in the 1932 film of the same name: "The Grand Hotel. Always the same. People come. People go . . . nothing ever happens."

A lot happened.

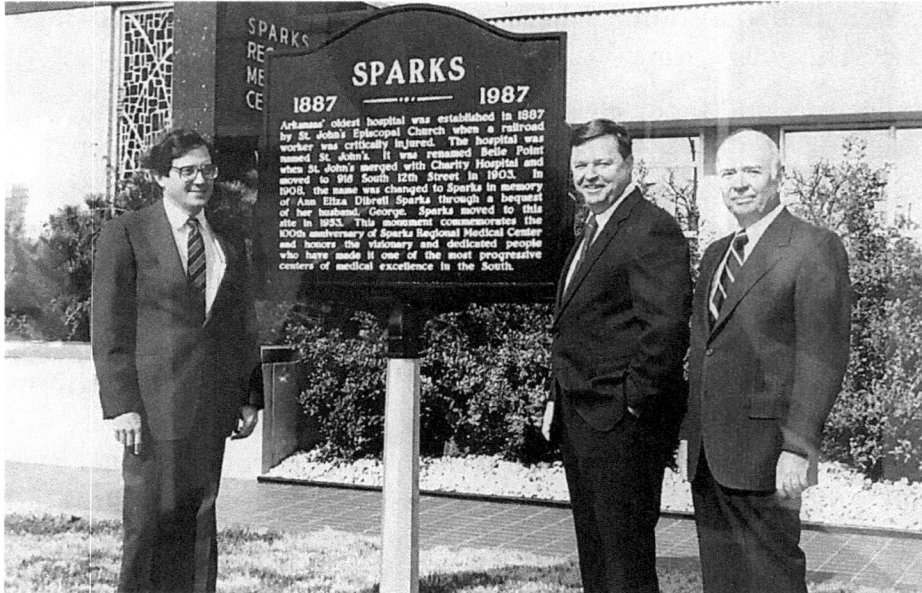

Charles Shuffield, chief executive officer of Sparks, on the left, stands by a plaque commemorating the one-hundred-year anniversary of the founding of Sparks Regional Medical Center in 1987. Robert A. Young, Jr., and Jim Alexander on the right, of the Sparks board of trustees, stand on the right. (Photo from Baptist Fort Smith archives)

Sparks became the largest hospital in Arkansas when it dedicated its six-level 206-bed east wing in 1979. [1] Several additions were made to the physical plant, but then in 2009 the non-profit community hospital was sold to a for-profit company, Health Management Associates (HMA), based in Naples, Florida. This transaction provided the wherewithal to fund the Arkansas College of Health Education

(ACHE), parent organization of the Arkansas College of Osteopathic Medicine and the College of Health Sciences. The Degen Foundation was created with some of the proceeds of the sale of Sparks to HMA, and this provided the initial ACHE funding to build the $32.4 million facility in the Chaffee Crossing area. [2] The osteopathic school admitted its first class in 2017.

And then in 2014 HMA sold Sparks to Community Health Systems (CHS), based in Franklin, Tennessee. Less than five years later Sparks changed hands for the third time in a decade and again became a non-profit hospital when Baptist Health System of Little Rock purchased it from CHS [3] and changed its name from Sparks to Baptist Health-Fort Smith.

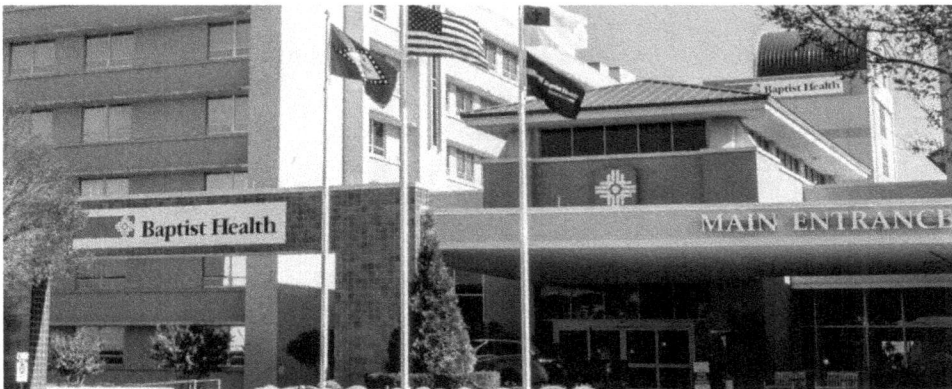

Main entrance to the Baptist Health hospital. (www.baptist-health.com/location/baptist-health-fort-smith)

Holt-Krock Clinic turned over its management to PhyCor, a Nashville-based management company, in 1992, making PhyCor the capital and managing partner for forty years. Doctors began leaving the clinic in 1998 over contract disputes, and PhyCor contended in a lawsuit against Sparks Hospital that more than sixty of the clinic's one hundred fifty-one physicians were leaving the clinic to go elsewhere or join Sparks Foundation. The result of a mediation session was that Sparks acquired the clinic in early 1999 and changed its name from Holt-Krock to Sparks Medical Foundation. [4]

Cooper Clinic, though never as large as Holt-Krock, expanded to as many as one hundred twenty-five physicians and moved from its Waldron Road location to a five-story building on the St. Edward campus in 1995. In time the relationship between clinic and hospital became adversarial. There was a lawsuit, but it was settled before an announcement in November 2017, that Cooper Clinic and Mercy would merge, with forty-eight Cooper Clinic physicians joining the Mercy network. [5] The Cooper Clinic name disappeared, as had that of Holt-Krock, and the building was renamed Mercy Tower West.

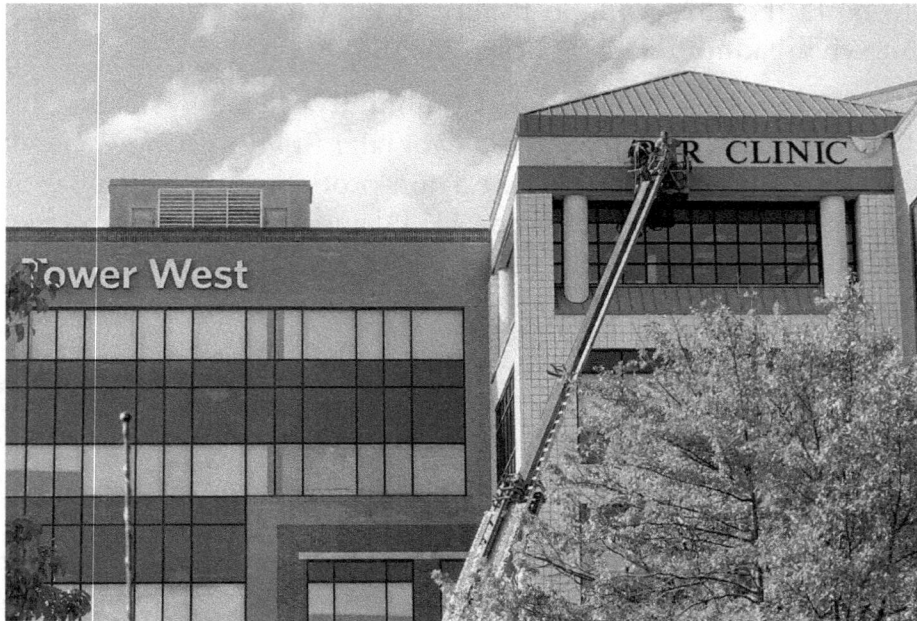

Changing the name of the building. (Photo by author)

The name St. Edward had already disappeared in 2012 as Mercy Health of St. Louis renamed all its hospitals Mercy.

The most recent figures, updated in June 2022, show that Mercy Fort Smith (including Mercy Orthopedic Hospital) has 256 staffed beds; there were 16,588 total discharges in a year and 75,255 patient days. [6] Baptist Health-Fort Smith has 321 staffed beds with 11,894 total discharges and 64,517 patient days. [7]

The inaugural class of 145 osteopathic medical students graduated from the Arkansas College of Osteopathic Medicine, located at Chaffee Crossing in Fort Smith, on May 15, 2021. Other facilities on the campus of the Arkansas Colleges of Health Education include the School of Physical Therapy and the School of Occupational Therapy. [8]

Clinics grow, and clinics die. Hospitals change their names, and one of them is sold three times. A new osteopathic college appears. People come. People go . . . nothing ever happens.

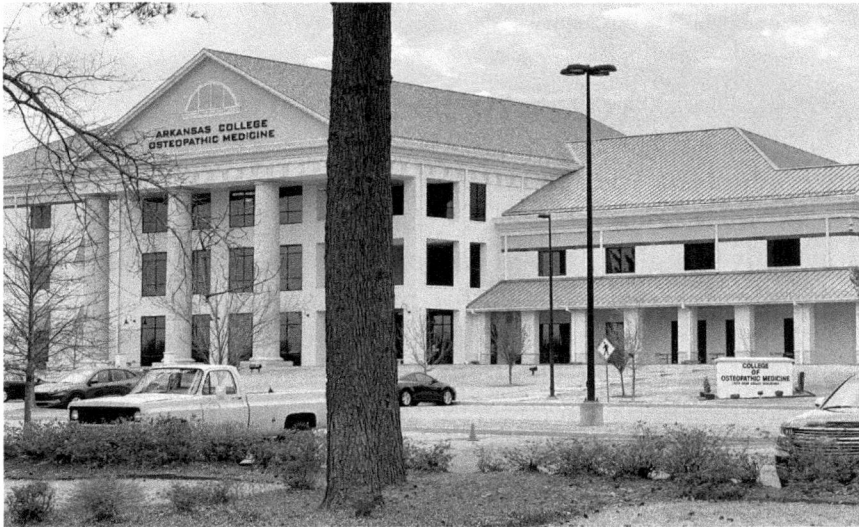

The Arkansas College of Osteopathic Medicine (Photo by author)

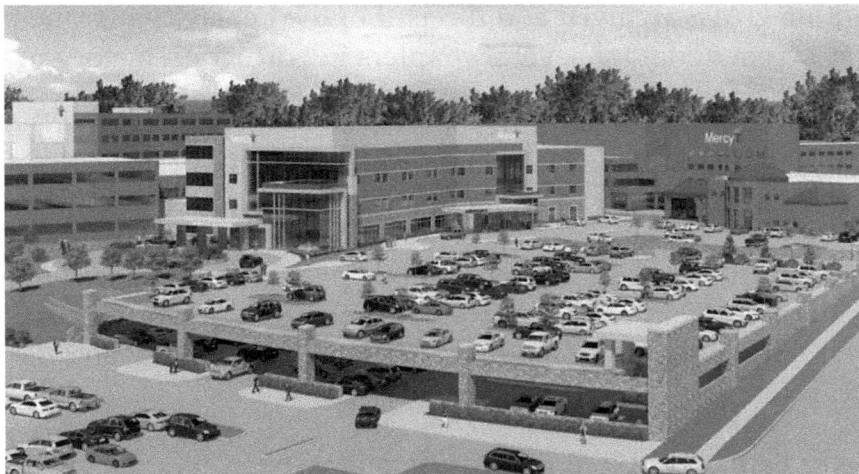

Mercy is expanding its emergency room, intensive care unit, and parking space, expected to open in late 2024. (www.mercy.net/newsroom/2021-06-30/mercy-hospital-fort-smith-announces)

Acknowledgments

Many of those who took time to talk to me about friends or family members are mentioned in the end notes of various chapters, but there were others whom I must mention. Billy Higgins, retired associated professor of history at University of Arkansas Fort Smith, served as editor of *The Journal of the Fort Smith Historical Society* during the time that many of these chapters appeared in the *Journal*; and his encouragement and advice with these chapters and then with assembling them into the nucleus of this book have been vital in bringing this work into the light of day. Thank you, Billy; you've helped make it fun to do.

Joe Wasson knows the history of Fort Smith as does no one else. I've consulted him and his wife Lynn as I've worked through the history of the area.

Shelley Blanton, UAFS archivist and director of the Pebley Center, helped greatly in tracking down material for several chapters in Fort Smith history.

Liz Haupert and her late mother Elizabeth Wolferman helped me for many years to feel like I knew Dr. Sidney Wolferman personally; and I had great fun sorting through a collection of family memorabilia with Liz.

Several other family members of those who appear in these pages have helped to provide memories, family photographs, memoirs, and memorabilia: Bob Hornberger, Harry Foltz, Cole Goodman, Virginia Bost Berner, and the late Sanna Olson Sullivan.

John and Joyce Faulkner of Red Engine Press have been generous with their time, patience, experience, and expertise in the process of publication.

My wife Mary and children Kendrick, Ellen, and Sally have encouraged me in my eccentricities; Mary proofreads everything that goes out of the house; Kendrick and Ellen, most of this material; and Ellen is the hands-on editor who can strip a chapter to its bare bones and help rebuild it. Thanks to you all for loving assistance.

Notes

The First Hundred Years

1   Amelia Martin, *Physicians and Medicine: Crawford and Sebastian Counties, Arkansas* (Fort Smith: Sebastian County Medical Society, 1977), 2-3.

2   Maranda Radcliff, "Fort Smith National Cemetery," *Encyclopedia of Arkansas History and Culture* https://encyclopediaofarkansas.net/entries/fort-smithnational-cemetery-2943. Accessed 9 Jan. 2014.

3   Russell was one of several doctors who at about that time came to the Territory of Arkansas, which was carved out of the Missouri Territory in 1819. Dr. Matthew Cunningham arrived at the site of Little Rock in early 1820 as the first physician there and served as Little Rock's first mayor. The names of ten other physicians appeared in various court records before 1821; the earliest mentioned was Dr. Robert Slaughter, who received a merchant's license at Arkansas Post in 1812, shortly after the Louisiana Territory was renamed the Missouri Territory (to avoid confusion with the newly created state of Louisiana, formed in 1812). By 1829 there were five doctors in Little Rock. Marion Stark Craig, "Doctors and Medicine in the Territory of Arkansas: 1819-1836," *An Anthology of Arkansas Medicine 1875-1975* (Arkansas Medical Society, 1975): 5-16.

4   Thomas Nuttall, *A Journal of Travels into the Arkansas Territory During the Year 1819*, ed. by Savoie Lottinville (Fayetteville: University of Arkansas Press, 1999), 237. Originally published Philadelphia, T. H. Palmer, 1821.

5   Martin, 8.

6   Martin, 11.

7   J. Fred Patton, *The History of Fort Smith 1817 through 2013* (North Little Rock, AR: Prestige Press, 7th ed., 2014), 74.

8   Martin, 12.

9   Odie B. Faulk and Billy Mac Jones, Fort Smith: *An Illustrated History* (Western Heritage Books, 1983), 191.

10 Angela Walton-Raji, "U. S. Military Hospital and Freedman's Hospital Fort Smith, Arkansas," *Journal of the Fort Smith Historical Society* 22, no. 2 (Sep. 1998): 19-20.

11 Walton-Raji, 19-20.

12 Martin, 29.

13 Martin, 55-56.

14 Martin, 55.

15 Arthur Hertzler, *The Horse and Buggy Doctor* (New York: Harper & Brothers, 1938), 247.

16   Lewis Thomas, *The Youngest Science: Notes of a Medicine-Watcher* (New York: Viking Press, 1983), 12-15.

17   W.B. Reid, "A Use of the Automobile in Surgical Practice, with Report of an Illustrative Case," *Am J Surg* 22, 2 (1908): 77-78.

18   Thomas, 12-15.

19   Henry Hollenberg, "Centennial Medical History of Little Rock and Central Arkansas," ed. by Horace N. Marvin, *An Anthology of Arkansas Medicine* (Arkansas Medical Society, 1975): 23.

20   Martin, 29-30.

21   Hertzler, 63.

22   Martin, 20-21.

23   Martin, 22.

24   Walton-Raji, 20.

25   Martin, 28.

26   Martin, 44.

27   Martin, 34.

28   Molly Crosby, The American Plague: *The Untold Story of Yellow Fever, the Epidemic that Shaped our History* (New York: The Berkley Publishing Group, 2007): 30-47.

29   Hollenberg, 23.

30   Michael Dougan, "Health and Medicine," *Encyclopedia of Arkansas History and Culture*, encyclopediaofarkansas.net/entries/health-and-medicine-392. Accessed 28 Dec. 2013.

31   Dougan, accessed November 18, 2019.

32   David Oshinsky, *Bellevue: Three Centuries of Medicine and Mayhem at America's Most Storied Hospital* (New York: Doubleday, 2016), 76.

33   Martin, 91.

34   Betty Battenfield, "Dr. James A. Dibrell, Sr.," *Arkansas Country Doctor Museum*, drmuseum.net/dr-james-a-dibrell-sr-2/. Accessed 13 Mar. 2023.

35   Battenfield, accessed 13 Mar. 2023.

36   Battenfield, accessed 13 Mar. 2023.

37   Oshinsky, 77.

38   Robert C. Watson, "Medicine's Contribution to Arkansas," *An Anthology of Arkansas Medicine 1875-1975*, (Arkansas Medical Society, 1975), 59.

39   Martin, 36.

40   Martin, 37-39.

41   Martin, 219-221.

42   Martin, 133-137.

43   Martin, 133.

44   Martin, 140.

45   Martin, 139.

46   Martin, 158,159, 451.

47   This description of the founding of the Catholic mission movement in Fort Smith
      and the subsequent founding of St. Edward's Infirmary is taken from Jane Ramos,
      *Arkansas Frontiers of Mercy: A History of the Sisters of Mercy in the Diocese of Little
      Rock* (St. Edward Press, 1989), and from Martin, *Physicians and Medicine*, 150-155.

48   Martin, 42-43.

49   Rutkow, I. *Seeking the Cure: A History of Medicine in America*. New York: Scribner,
      2010: 181.

50   Rutkow, 67.

51   Martin, 43.

52   Martin, 50-51.

The Legendary Smiths and Their Paris Hospital

Dr. John Charles Smith was one of the co-authors of an earlier version of this
chapter published in the *Journal of the Arkansas Medical Society* in 2013, and he
provided much information from his personal recollections of family stories;
several further anecdotes were collected by Earl and Glenda Schrock in an
unpublished family history written in 1994.

1   Earl and Glenda Schrock, *Doctors All: The Descendants of Arthur F. Smith in Western
     Arkansas* (Published privately for Smith family, 1994), 4.

2   Schrock, 17.

3   Zackery A Cothren, "Arkansas Listings in the National Register of Historic Places:
     Hospitals," *The Arkansas Historical Quarterly* 64, no. 4 (2005): 425-430.

4   Schrock, 45.

5   Amelia Martin, *Physicians and Medicine: Crawford and Sebastian Counties, Arkansas*
     (Fort Smith: Sebastian County Medical Society, 1977), 162.

6   *The Encyclopedia of Arkansas History and Culture: Paris (Logan County)*. http://
     www.encyclopediaofarkansas.net/encyclopedia/entry-
     detail.aspx?entryID=924. Accessed 27 Nov. 2013.

7   Schrock, 59-61.

8   Schrock, 62.

9   Schrock, 122-123.

10 Jo Ann B. Miller, "The Florence Nightingales of the Hospital-on-the-Hill: Part 1 on Nurses at the Paris (Smith) Hospital," *Wagon Wheels* (Journal of the Logan County Historical Society), 1997f: 15-21.

11 Schrock, 160.

The Doctor and the Mastodon

1 "A Mastodon Found in Arkansas," *New York Times*, 15 Nov. 1885.

2 Amelia Martin, *Physicians and Medicine: Crawford and Sebastian Counties, Arkansas 1817-1976* (Fort Smith, published by Sebastian County Medical Society, 1977), 248-249.

3 James Tichgelaar, *Crowley's Ridge Mastodon* (Arkansas State University Museum booklet, undated).

4 "Molar of a Mastodon," *Arkansas Gazette*, 16 Apr. 1890.

5 "Fossil Friday, A Fossil of not Quite Mammoth Proportions," *Paleoaerie: Arkansas Educational Resource Initiative for Evolution and Arkansas Paleontology* paleoaerie.org/2014/02/07/fossil-friday-a-fossil-of-not-quite-mammothproportions/. Accessed 17 Sep. 2023.

6 "Permanent Exhibits," *Mid America Science Museum*, midamericamuseum.org/exhibits/permanent-exhibits/. Accessed 17 Sep. 2023.

7 "Island 35 Mastodon," *Wikipedia*, www.wikiwand.com/en/Island_35_Mastodon. Accessed 17 Sep. 2023.

8 John Surratt, "Bovina Youth Find Buried Mastodon Jaw," *The Vicksburg Post*, 19 Mar. 2018 https://www.vicksburgpost.com/2018/03/19/bovina-youth-findburied- mastodon. Accessed 17 Sep. 2023.

9 Paul Semonen, *American Monster: How the Nation's First Prehistoric Creature Became a Symbol of National Identity* (New York: New York University Press, 2000), 3.

10 Semonen, 42.

11 Elizabeth Kolbert, *The Sixth Extinction: An Unnatural History* (Henry Holt and Co., 2014), 36.

12 Martin, 250.

13 The Encyclopedia of the New West, Edited by William S. Speer and John Henry Brown (United States Biographical Publishing Company, 1881), Arkansas, 35-36.).

14 "87 Years Young, Still Practicing Medicine," *Arkansas Gazette*, 1 Sep. 1912.

15 "Pioneer Physician Dies at Van Buren," *Arkansas Gazette*, 24 Apr. 1913.

16 *History of Benton, Washington, Carroll, Madison, Crawford, Franklin, and Sebastian Counties, Arkansas*, (Higginson Book Company, 1889) 588.

When the Flu Hit Home

1   *Southwest American*, 10 Oct. 1918.

2   *Southwest American*, 2 Nov. 1918.

3   *Arkansas Gazette*, 2 Nov. 1918 (provided by Dr. Joseph H. Bates, Associate Dean for Public Health Practice, University of Arkansas for Medical Sciences).

4   Steven Teske, "World War I," *CALS Encyclopedia of Arkansas* encyclopediaofarkansas.net/encyclopedia/entry-detail.aspx?entryID=2401. Accessed 30 Apr. 2019.

5   Carol Byerly, "War Losses (USA)" *1914-1918-online. International Encyclopedia of the First World War* encyclopedia.1914-1918-online.net/article/war_losses_usa. Accessed 30 Apr. 2019.

6   "Spanish Flu," *History* https://www.history.com/topics/world-war-i/1918-flupandemic. Accessed 17 Sep. 2023.

7   Fred Patton, *The History of Fort Smith 1817 through 2013* (North Little Rock, AR: Prestige Press, 7th ed., 2014).

8   K.A. Scott, "Plague on the Homefront: Arkansas and the Great Influenza Epidemic of 1918," *Arkansas Historical Quarterly* 47, no. 4, 1988: 311-344.

9   John M. Barry, *The Great Influenza: The Epic Story of the Deadliest Plague in Human History* (New York: Viking Press, 2004), 216-217.

10 Nancy Hendricks, "PLAGUE: The 1918 Influenza Epidemic in Arkansas." *To Can the Kaiser: Arkansas and the Great War*, ed. by Michael D. Polston and Guy Lancaster (Little Rock: Butler Center Books, 2015), 137.

11 Jack Schnedler, "Death grippe: The Other Great War in 1918 — Against Influenza — Killed Millions Globally and Thousands Locally," *Arkansas Gazette*, 24 Sep. 2018.

12 Scott, 321.

13 Scott, 317.

14 "Proclamation," *Southwest American*, 9 Oct. 1918

15 "A Plea for Volunteers to Assist in Nursing," *Southwest American*, 8 Oct. 1918.

16 Barry, 320.

17 Barry, 351.

18 Barry, 242.

19 Barry, 187-188.

20 *Southwest American*, Oct. 1918.

21 "19 DIE OF INFLUENZA: Cases at Fort Smith Decrease and Situation is Improved," *Arkansas Gazette*, 16 Oct. 1918.

22 "5 Deaths at Ft. Smith: Is Largest One-Day Toll Since Influenza Epidemic Began," *Arkansas Gazette,* 18 Oct. 1918.

23 Personal communications to author, Matthew Hicks, Sebastian County Health Unit Administrator, 13 Feb. 2019, and Dirk Haselow, State Epidemiologist, Arkansas Department of Health, 14 Feb. 2019.

24 Scott, 320.

25 "Death Rate Low from Disease Here," *Southwest American,* 20 Oct. 1918.

26 Personal communication to author, Mike Dewitt, 17 Mar. 2019.

27 Amelia Martin, *Physicians and Medicine: Crawford and Sebastian Counties, Arkansas 1817-1976* (Fort Smith: Sebastian County Medical Society, 1977), 61.

28 Martin, 635.

29 Martin, 502.

30 Martin, 444.

31 Carolyn Gray LeMaster, *A Corner Of The Tapestry: A History Of The Jewish Experience In Arkansas, 1820s – 1990s* (Fayetteville: The University of Arkansas Press, 1994), 217.

32 Cathy Boyd, "Ben Drew Kimpel (1915-1983)," *CALS Encyclopedia of Arkansas* encyclopediaofarkansas.net/entries/ben-drew-kimpel-1688/. Accessed 16 Mar. 2019.

33 "Biography: Victor Vaughn." PBS. An American Experience https://www.pbs.org/wgbh/americanexperience/features/influenza-victor-vaughan/. Accessed 16 Mar. 2019.

34 Barry, 391.

35 Barry, 391.

36 Barry, 392.

37 Scott, 332.

38 "Morris-Morton Drug Co.—Fort Smith AR." Waymark.waymarking.com/waymarks/WMN7WW_Morris_Morton_Drug_Co_Fort_Smith_AR. Accessed 30 Apr. 2019.

39 Scott, 337.

40 "Tulsa Race Massacre," *Wikipedia* en.wikipedia.org/wiki/Tulsa_race_massacre. Accessed 16 Mar. 2019.

41 "Elaine Massacre," *Wikipedia* en.wikipedia.org /wiki/Elainemassacre. Accessed 16 Mar. 2019.

Founding Fathers

Dr. Fred Krock's younger son, Dr. Curtis Krock, is an old friend who was in practice at Holt-Krock Clinic during my first three years in Fort Smith. He has provided much helpful information about his father and Holt-Krock Clinic, along with some excellent photographs.

Joseph St. Cloud Irwin has been in contact with the Cooper family about the Cooper history, and he has provided interesting bits of family history, with some photographs I had not previously seen.

Several cardboard boxes of papers, photographs, artifacts, and other memorabilia have been saved in Cooper Clinic for years. The Cooper, Wolferman, and Goldstein families have donated family items to this collection.

The late Amelia Martin's comprehensive history, *Physicians and Medicine: Crawford and Sebastian Counties, Arkansas 1817-1976* (1977) continues to be an invaluable source of detailed information.

When not otherwise noted below, these four sources have provided background information for this paper.

1   Odie B. Faulk and Billy Mac Jones, *Fort Smith: An Illustrated History* (Muskogee, Western Heritage Books, 1983)195.

2   Notes in Cooper Clinic archives.

3   "Doctor Fails to Rally from Heart Attack," *Southwest American*, 23 Mar. 1930.

4   D. Musgrove, "Dr. Charles S. Holt," *Country Doctors of Sebastian County*, argenweb.net/sebastian/Doctors/Doctors.html. Accessed 25 Sep. 2023.

5   Amelia Martin, *Physicians and Medicine: Crawford and Sebastian Counties, Arkansas 1817-1976* (Fort Smith, Published by Sebastian County Medical Society, 1977) 158-160.

6   Josie Decker, "Holt-Krock Clinic 1921-1999," *The Journal of the Fort Smith Historical Society*, 26 (April 2002) 2-7.

7   Decker, 6.

8   "Dr. Holt to Manage Sparks Hospital," *Southwest American*, 3 Apr. 1934.

9   Personal communication to author, Curtis Krock. Accessed 4 Feb. 2018

Present at the Creation

1   Taylor Prewitt, "Founding Fathers: St. Cloud Cooper, Charles Holt, and Fred Krock, and their Innovative Clinics," *The Journal of the Fort Smith Historical Society*, 42, 1 (April 2018), 5-12.

2   Personal interview by author with Irvin Sternberg.

3   Personal interview by author with Liz Wolferman Haupert.

4   Amelia Martin, *Physicians and Medicine: Crawford and Sebastian Counties, Arkansas 1817-1976* (Fort Smith: Sebastian County Medical Society, 1977), 338-339.

5   Cooper Clinic minutes, 1920, from archives, Pebley Center, University of Arkansas-Fort Smith.

6   J. Kenneth Thompson, "History of the Cooper Clinic," talk delivered at 70th Anniversary dinner, Fort Smith, 7 Apr. 1990.

7   *Journal of Arkansas Medical Society* 7, 1933.

8   Thompson, 1990.

9   *Daily Herald*, Fort Smith Ark. 26 Sep. 1912 (clipping provided by Pebley Center, UAFS).

10   *Daily Herald*, Fort Smith Ark. 10 Jul. 1913 (clipping provided by Pebley Center, UAFS).

11   Julia Yadon, Sue Ross Cross, Randall Ross Viguet, *Reflections of Fort Smith* (Fort Smith: Fort Smith Historical Press. 1978), 101.

12   Thompson, 1990.

13   Martin, 339.

14   Personal interview by author with Liz Wolferman Haupert, 8 Sep. 2018.

15   "Insane from High Prices: Expert Says Cost of Living Unbalances Minds," *New York World*, 7 Feb. 1913.

16   Clipping from unknown publication, in family collection of Elizabeth Wolferman Haupert, 24 Jan. 1917.

17   Haupert collection, 5 Apr. 1917.

18   "High Honor for Dr. Wolferman: Chosen from Ft. Smith to Specialize in Surgery," *The Independent-Times*, Streator, IL, undated, in family collection of Elizabeth Wolferman Haupert.

19   Martin, 634.

20   Cooper Clinic archives, Pebley Center, University of Arkansas-Fort Smith.

21   Cooper Clinic archives, Pebley Center, University of Arkansas-Fort Smith.

22   Cooper Clinic archives, Pebley Center, University of Arkansas-Fort Smith.

23   Cooper Clinic archives, Pebley Center, University of Arkansas-Fort Smith.

24   Thompson, 1990.

25   Carolyn LeMaster, *A Corner of the Tapestry: A History of the Jewish Experience in Arkansas*, 1820s-1990s. (Fayetteville: University of Arkansas Press, 1994), 216.

26   Hollace Weiner, Mark Bauman, and BerkleyKalin, *The Quiet Voices: Southern Rabbis and Black Civil Rights, 1880s to 1990s*, ed. by Mark Bauman and Berkley Kalin. (Tuscaloosa: University of Alabama Press, 1997).

27   Thompson, 1990.

28   Thompson, 1990.

29   Martin, 353.

30   LeMaster, 453.

31   Martin, 241

32   Cooper Clinic archives, Pebley Center, University of Arkansas-Fort Smith

33   Martin, 241

34   Thompson, 1990.

A Breath of Fresh Air

1   Nancy Griffith, "Tuberculosis," *CALS Encyclopedia of Arkansas.* encyclopediaofarkansas.net/entries/tuberculosis-6439/. Accessed 18 Dec. 2019.

2   William Leeper, "Arkansas State Tuberculosis Sanatorium," *CALS Encyclopedia of Arkansas.* encyclopediaofarkansas.net/entries/arkansas-state-tuberculosissanatorium- 2237/. Accessed 19 Sep. 2019.

3   Personal communication with author, Joe Bates, 20 Apr. 2019.

4   Griffith, Accessed 19 Sep. 2019.

5   Griffith, Accessed 19 Sep. 2019.

6   "Committee will Study Offer of Wild Cat Mountain Camp," *Arkansas Gazette.* 2 Jan. 1937.

7   Amelia Martin, "Arkansas Tuberculosis Sanatorium Wildcat Mountain Annex," *The Journal of the Sebastian County Historical Society* 21:2 (1997), 12-14.

8   Personal communication with author, Joe S. Irwin, 2017.

9   Patsy Gadberry, "Leo Everett Nybeg," *Find a Grave.* .findagrave.com/ memorial/107061734/leo-everett-nyberg . Accessed 19 Dec. 2019.

10   Sven Peterson, "Arkansas State Tuberculosis Sanatorium: The Nation's Largest," *Arkansas Historical Quarterly* 5 (Winter 1946): 312–329.

11   David Koon, "Every Day was a Tuesday," *Arkansas Times* 17 Jun. 2010 arktimes.com/news/cover-stories/2010/06/17/every-day-was-a-tuesday? oid=1205540. Accessed 17 Jun. 2016.

12   Laverne Nelson, "A Personal View of a Young Woman's 'Time on the Hill': Arkansas Tuberculosis Sanatorium Booneville and Fort Smith," *The Journal of the Fort Smith Historical Society* 21 (2): 16-19, Sep., 1991

13   Joe Bates, W. E., Potts, M. Lewis, "Epidemiology of Tuberculosis in an Industrial School," *New England Journal of Medicine* 272, no. 14, 1965, 714-717.

14   Leeper, Accessed 10 Sep. 2019.

15   Sam Taggart. *The Public's Health: A Narrative History of Health and Disease in Arkansas* (Little Rock: Arkansas Times Press, 2013), 75.

16   "How Dr. Joe Bates changed the face of Tuberculosis," achi.net/library/dr-batestuberculosis- treatment/. Accessed 19 Dec. 2019.

17   Leeper, Accessed 19 Sep. 2019.

18   Billy D. Higgins, Stephen Husarik, and Henry Q. Rinne, *University of Arkansas-Fort Smith: The First 85 Years* (USA: RPR Book Group, 2012), 34.

19   Martin, 12.

20   "Home Dedication Scheduled Today". *Arkansas Gazette* 1 Mar. 1961.

21   Leeper, Accessed 7 Oct. 2019.

22   "The Sanatorium Files. Part 3—The Sanatorium Movement," *Working Group on New TB Drugs* newtbdrugs.org/news/sanatorium-files-part-3—-sanatoriummovement. Accessed 25 Sep. 2023.

23   William W. Stead, "Tuberculosis." *In Harrison's Principles of Internal Medicine*, 6th ed., edited by Maxwell M. Wintrobe et al, 866. New York: McGraw-Hill Co., 1970.

24   "Tuberculosis (TB): Data and Statistics, *CDC* cdc.gov/tb/statistics/default.htm. Accessed 30 Sep. 2019.

25   David Bulit, "A. G. Holley State Hospital," *Abandoned FL* abandonedfl.com/a-gholley- state-hospital. Accessed 28 Sep. 2019.

Postwar Renaissance

I had the good fortune to know personally the doctors described in this chapter, and much of the material presented is based on my own recollections and, rather heavily, on the recollections of their sons and daughters, who are named in the Acknowledgements. Many details of their backgrounds are taken from Amelia Martin's *Physicians and Medicine: Crawford and Sebastian Counties, Arkansas 1817-1976* (Fort Smith, published by Sebastian County Medical Society, 1977).

1   Odie B. Faulk and Billy Mac Jones, *Fort Smith: An Illustrated History*, (Muskogee: Western Heritage Books, 1983), 220.

2   J. Kenneth Thompson, "History of the Cooper Clinic," talk delivered at 70th Anniversary dinner, Fort Smith, 7 Apr. 1990.

He Knew Who He Was

Although standard practice is to refer to people by their surname after first identification gives both given name and surname, I have sometimes referred to Harry McDonald as "Dr. McDonald" and sometimes by his first name only, sometimes to avoid confusion with other family members, and sometimes because of the context.

Maria McDonald McNamar, Palmer McDonald, Euba Winton, George McGill, and Charlotte Tidwell have been most helpful and patient in sharing with me their recollections of Dr. McDonald. Dr. McDonald's own recollections have also been used extensively. Major attributions are so noted in the bibliography, but to avoid an even more lengthy list of references, some minor attributions have been omitted. Unless otherwise noted, information for this work has come from one of these five people or from Dr. McDonald's own quotations.

A personal addendum: It was a surprise to find my own name mentioned by Dr. McDonald in the transcript of a 2001 interview, in which he listed me among three physicians in Fort Smith who were "willing to see his patients, take his calls, and work with him." I certainly did, and it was always an honor for me to see any of Dr. McDonald's patients.

1   Personal communication to author, George McGill, 2017.

2   John A. Kirk, "'Please Help Us': The Fort Smith Congress of Racial Equality Chapter, 1962-1965," *Arkansas Historical Quarterly* 73, no.3, 2014: 293-317.

3   Personal communication to author, Randolph Ney, 2017.

4   Personal communication to author, Charlotte Tidwell, 2017

5   "Fort Smith Board Ordered to Integrate City's High Schools," *Arkansas Gazette*, 7 Dec. 1965, on file in Pebley Center, University of Arkansas-Fort Smith.

6   Coretta King, Letter to Harry McDonald, 29 May 1969.

7   Personal communication to author, Palmer McDonald, 2017.

8   Personal communication to author, Euba Winton, 2017.

9   Personal communication to author, Palmer McDonald, 2017.

10 Personal communication to author, Palmer McDonald, 2017.

11 Cynthia Howell, "Fort Smith's Only Black Doctor Leaving his Mark," *Arkansas Democrat*, 2 July 1990.

12 Harry McDonald, Telephone interview, 4 May 2001, on file in Pebley Center, University of Arkansas-Fort Smith.

13 Jennifer Shields, "Outspoken Activist Retiring," *Southwest Times Record*, 17 Aug. 1990.

14 McGill, 2017.

15 Howell, 1990.

16 Amanda Sturgill, "Sumter Native Has Led a Full Life of Healing, Helping, and Changing," *The Sumter (South Carolina) Item*, 30 Nov. 1990.

17 "City Renames Local Park After Martin Luther King," *Fort Smith Times Record*, 22 Apr. 1969.

18 McDonald, 2001.

19 McDonald, 2001.

20 *Lincoln High School History*, ed. by Sherry Toliver and Barbara Webster-Meadows, (published 2014), 297.

21 Personal communication to author, Maria McDonald McNamar, 2017.

Ninety Percent Backbone

1   "Dr. Roger Browning Bost 1921-2013," Legacy, legacy.com/obituaries/batesville/name/ dr-roger-bost-obituary?id=7008833. Accessed 30 Nov. 2022.

2   Nate Hinkel, "Historical Diploma, Photos Donated to College of Pharmacy," *UAMS News*, 2010.

3   "Roger Browning Bost," *crunchbase*, .crunchbase.com/person/roger-browning-bost, Accessed 20 Nov. 2022.

4   "Bost Inc. Founder Dr. Roger Bost Dies At 92," *Fort Smith Times Record*, 18 Nov. 2013.

5   Dwain Hebda, "Simply the Bost," *Do South Magazine*, 2020.

6   Ernest Dumas, "Roger Bost, Children's Champion," *Arkansas Times*, 28 Nov. 2013.

7   Dumas, 2013.

Epilogue

1   Kevin Laval: "Sparks: New patient wing dedicated," *Southwest Times Record*, 17 Sep. 1979.

2   Michael Tilley, "Sparks Health in Fort Smith, Van Buren sold to Little Rock-based Baptist Health," *TB&P* 18 Jul., talkbusiness.net/2018/07/sparks-health-in-fort-smith- van-buren-sold-to-little-rock-based-baptist-health/. Accessed 30 Sep. 2019.

3   Tilly, 2018.

4   Jose Decker, "Holt Krock Clinic 1921-1999," *Journal of the Fort Smith Historical Society*, 26 no. 1 (April 2002), 2-7.

5   "48 Cooper Clinic doctors now part of Mercy Clinic-Fort Smith," TB&P 1 Nov. 2017, talkbusiness.net/2017/11/48-cooper-clinic-doctors-now-part-of-mercy-clinic-fort-smith/. Accessed 1 Oct. 2019.

6   *American Hospital Directory*, ahd.com/free_profile/040062/ Mercy_Hospital_Fort_Smith/ Fort_Smith/Arkansas/. Accessed 7 Mar. 2023.

7   *American Hospital Directory*, ahd.com/free_profile/040055/Baptist_Health-Fort_Smith/Fort_Smith/Arkansas/. Accessed 7 Mar. 2023.

8   "About ACHE," *Arkansas Colleges of Health and Education*, achehealth.edu/ about. Accessed 7 Mar. 2023.

About the Author

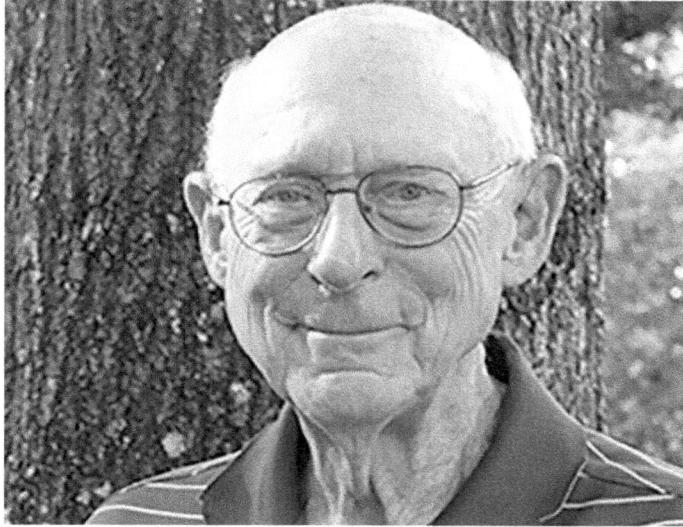

Taylor Prewitt, a retired cardiologist, has published papers on the history of medicine in *The Journal of the Fort Smith Historical Society* and *The Journal of the Arkansas Medical Society* for the past ten years. These papers form the nucleus of *Before It Got Complicated: Medicine in Fort Smith and the Arkansas River Valley 1817-1975*. He received the Walter L. Brown Award for Best Biography, Autobiography, or Memoir in a county or local journal in 2018 for "'He Knew Who He Was:' Reflections on the Life of Harry P. McDonald."

Prewitt grew up in McGehee, Arkansas; majored in English at the University of Arkansas; graduated from Washington University School of Medicine in St. Louis; and trained in cardiology at the University of North Carolina in Chapel Hill. He practiced at Cooper Clinic in Fort Smith from 1969 to 2003, also serving as a senior fellow in cardiology at the Brompton Hospital in London during the year 1974. Among other professional recognition, he is a Master of the American College of Physicians.

His books include *Reciting Robert Frost in the ICU: Essays on the Literature of Medicine* and most recently, a collection of personal essays and book reviews, *Notes in the Margin: Reflections on a Few Books* in 2022. He also spoke to the Trollope Society in

New York about his book *The Way They Lived Then: Serious Interviews, Strong Women, and Lessons for Life in the Novels of Anthony Trollope*. He and his wife Mary live in Fort Smith. They have three children and seven grandchildren. Other interests include swimming, tennis, and photography.

www.ingramcontent.com/pod-product-compliance
Lightning Source LLC
Chambersburg PA
CBHW080645270326
41928CB00017B/3197